# Stolen Money, Stolen Health

## A Surgeon/Minister's Practical Reasons for Healthcare Reform

Rev. Lydell C. Lettsome, MD, FACS

First Printing, 2014

# Contents

# Dedication

To the Honorable William H. Gray, III and George M. Ross, the co-founders of Operation Understanding, for creating a program that has inspired hundreds of youth to engage in civic discourse and leadership.

# Acknowledgements

Thank you to Almighty God for this amazing life that I'm allowed to live.

Thank you to my mother, Laris Lettsome, and my aunt, Dorcas Young, for constantly encouraging me to seek knowledge if for no other reason than truth.

Thank you to Professor Gary Dorrien for telling me that my voice was one that needed to be part of the public discourse on healthcare.

Thank you to my editors, fact checker and proof readers for their advice, support and editing.

Thank you to Donnie Light of eBook76 publishing and Gary McCluskey, Alexandra Uth and Rebecca Winters for their help with the final touches.

Thank you to my wife, Raquel, for believing in me, reading my many manuscripts, and encouraging me that this book is needed.

# Prologue

## *Obamacare Is Only a Small First Step*

In the fall of 2005, I met Olivia Grayson. She was a fifty-nine-year-old Caribbean American whom I was treating for stage II breast cancer. She had been living in the United States for more than 10 years and was a documented alien through the U.S. Department of Immigration with a steady job. Unfortunately, Ms. Grayson's job as a live-in domestic did not provide health insurance. Over the course of her treatment, I learned she did not qualify for emergency Medicaid Insurance because of her immigration status. We were eventually able to get Ms. Grayson financial assistance for her chemotherapy through a Catholic charity.

As a young surgeon barely two years into practicing medicine, I thought her sad scenario was uncommon and mainly due to her immigration status. However, I quickly learned there were many American citizens who were uninsured or underinsured for reasons having nothing to do with their immigration status. Millions of my fellow citizens work steady, low paying jobs with minimal benefits that make health care a luxury.

For years we have been told that limited and unequal access to health care exists mainly because of exorbitant costs. Indeed health care in America costs more than any other country. However, there is also more money available in the American health care system than any other country in the world. What many Americans do not know is that corporate executives are constantly siphoning off the money.

The Patient Protection and Affordable Care Act (PPACA), a brainchild of the Obama Administration, is actually based on previous Republican health care policies and is not a perfect law. But as both a doctor and cleric, I firmly believe the Affordable Care Act's ethos and intent are right and that it is fair. The PPACA returns some power to the people. It gives us leverage. It lets our voice be heard in an essential area of American life, one where the public has long been silenced.

Certainly, the opponents of the PPACA are correct in arguing that "Obamacare" affects individual rights and the flow of money throughout the gargantuan United States medical economy, which is huge and growing. But, with the PPACA, millions of Americans and small businesses will gain far more consumer rights, protection, and save money when it comes to their own health care. The PPACA is an initial step in what should be a much broader program of health care reform in the only leading, industrialized nation on Earth where some citizens still think it acceptable for other citizens to have no health care coverage at all.

Nonetheless, let me be clear. This book is not an Obamacare pamphlet in disguise. Nor do I feel that Obamacare is the ultimate answer. This book makes the argument that American health care suffers from the lack of true financial transparency, accountable moral standards, completeness of services, and decent customer service.

Indeed, it's a sad fact, that complex industry terminology and inflammatory media sound-bites make our eyes glaze over or tempers flare, preventing any meaningful dialogue about health reform. But let's not give in to imagined terrors and uncivility. We have got work to do. There is an ethical, medical, and fiscal obligation to forge ahead and create a health care system that benefits all and not just the fortunate ones, an idea that is firmly in line with the mandates of the United States Constitution.

As you read this book I hope to make it abundantly clear that assuring everyone gets good, affordable medicine and preventive care does not necessitate a whittling back of coverage or quality. Nor will it expose our economy to socialism or fiscal ruin.

# Chapter 1

## *The Urgency of Expansive Reform*

In 1994, when I was a second-year medical student, spending on health care accounted for approximately 14 percent of our nation's gross domestic product.[1] I was totally enthralled by the mere idea of joining a profession that was such a key driver of the U.S. economy.

But that excitement, which marked both my ignorance and my naïve motives, was short-lived. As I have pressed more fully into my career as a surgeon, it has become emphatically clear to me—and to a growing chorus of economists and medical analysts—that unrelenting increases in health care spending are going to bankrupt our economy. And this spending will leave our nation sicker and more medically unattended than we are right now.

My worries about what is at risk are shared by an array of medical clinicians, medical ethicists, scholars, advocates in daily contact with the uninsured, patients, and health providers in communities where hospitals and medical practices are shutting down. In a March 2012 New York Times article, Victor Fuchs Ph.D., a Stanford University professor emeritus of economics, health research and policy, said the record-breaking pace of health care spending was unduly burdening taxpayers and government resources: "Approximately fifty percent of

---

[1] KR Levitt, HC Lazenby, L Siverajan, "Health Care Spending I 1994: Slowest in Decades", Health Affairs; May 1996, p. 130-144; online at: http://content.healthaffairs.org/content/15/2/130 (accessed July 21, 2014)

all health care spending is now government spending. At the state and local level it is crowding out education, crowding out maintenance and repair of bridges and roads." [2]

Truly, in communities where schools are crumbling, 911 call response times are life-threateningly slow, and even the bridges and roads are deteriorating, health care costs are very much a part of the problem. That is true even if we do not, in our everyday thinking, precisely link health care spending to maintenance of municipal infrastructure and 911 rescues. Former New York City mayor, Michael Bloomberg, argued during the height of national debate over Obamacare that police and firefighters would have to pay more of their health insurance costs. Wal-Mart balked at providing health care coverage for its army of workers because in excess of 12% of employer payroll spending goes toward health care costs alone. In 2010, the Kaiser Family Foundation, a nonprofit health policy research group found that the median cost for health care was 12.8% of payroll.[3] This means there were just as many employers who spent less than that as those who spent more. A full-time job, paying $70,000 a year, can cost an employer an additional $12,000 to $17,000, on average, in health care insurance benefits alone. Concerned about their own profit margins and employee satisfaction with take-home pay, more employers are offering part-time jobs with zero benefits. The U.S. Bureau of Labor Statistics reported in May 2012 that the national tally of part-time jobs, defined as positions

---

[2] Kolata, Gina, "Knotty Challenges in Health Care Costs", New York Times, March 6, 2012; online at: http://www.nytimes.com/2012/03/06/healthpolicy/an-interview-with-victor-fuchs-on-health-care-costs.html?_r=0 (accessed July 21,2014)

[3] Gary Claxton and Anthony Damico, "Snapshots, Employer Health Insurance Costa and Worker Compensation," The Henry J. Kaiser Family Foundation, February 27, 2011;online at: http://kff.org/health-costs/issue-brief/snapshots-employer-health-insurance-costs-and-worker-compensation/ (accessed July 21, 2014)

requiring thirty-five or fewer hours of work each week, was at an all-time high.[4]

For the last 30 years, we have been embroiled in some variation of the present political and fiscal debate over the impact of health care expenditures in the workplace. We have debated what health care should cost and our very model of health care delivery, including what it does well and what it does quite poorly. A veritable cottage industry of analysts, commentators, and experts has sprouted up around the subject of health care policy.

We also have come up with a flurry of constructs for churning out health care. In the 1980s, managed care was the big thing. The latest model is Accountable Care Organizations[5], which links hospital and doctor payments to the quality of patient management and health outcomes.

However, most Americans do not have a clue about how this complicated and often frightening system really works. Most Americans do not understand the nuts-and-bolts. A February 2011 poll by the Kaiser Family Foundation showed that almost a year after the Affordable Care Act became law, only 52% of Americans even knew that it existed, let alone what it provided.[6] This *lack of awareness* is part of what brings us to this urgent hour; an hour when governors in twenty-three states have refused to participate in Obamacare's

[4] U.S. Bureau of Labor Statistics, Labor Force Survey, 2012;online at:
http://www.census.gov.ph/old/data/pressrelease/2012/lf1204tx.html (accessed July 24, 2014)
[5] Centers for Medicare and Medicaid, Shared Savings Program Brief, ;online at:
http://www.cms.gov/Medicare/Medicare-Fee-for-Service-Payment/sharedsavingsprogram/Index.html?redirect=/sharedsavingsprogram/ (accessed July 21, 2014)
[6] Kaiser Family Foundation, "Health Reform Poll Finding", Henry J. Kaiser Family Foundation; online at:
http//kaiserfamilyfoundation.files.wordpress.com/2013/01/8156-f.pdf (accessed July 21, 2014)

Medicaid expansion, which is the main vehicle for extending coverage to the working-poor people who are without insurance. As we examine the work of reforming health care that Obamacare only begins to address, we cannot ignore the details. We must have an informed, civil discussion about how to move forward, spending only what is necessary on health care, while creating a system that produces far better results. We must move the United States, a global power and pacesetter, out of last place in the health care rankings.

**According to a 2010 study by the nonprofit Commonwealth Fund, the U.S. was ranked number seven in health outcomes among seven leading industrialized nations.** [7] In the World Health Organization's 2000 ranking of health outcomes for 194 countries, the U.S. came in 37th place.[8]

The blueprint for fixing what ails American health care is revealed in the following pages and based upon my own intensive research. I have mined medical studies and white papers by health care companies and foundations, pharmaceutical firms, and advocacy groups on both the left and right including but not limited to Milliman Inc., Deloitte Consulting, the Kaiser Family Foundation, Healthcare-NOW, the Commonwealth Fund, and the Robert Wood Johnson Foundation. I have had long talks with colleagues in my dual fields of medicine and Christian ministry who also are concerned about the trajectory we are on. In no small measure, my everyday conversations with patients, friends, and relatives about their various encounters with our health care system also shape this blueprint.

---

[7] U.S. Ranks Last Among Seven Countries Health System Performance Measures, Commonwealth Fund.org,  Briefs, June 25 Issue, http://www.commonwealthfund.org/publications/newsletters/the-commonwealth-fund-connection/2010/june-25-2010, (accessed July 21, 2014)

[8] Christopher J.L. Murray and Julio Frank, "Ranking 37th-Measuring the Performance of the U.S. Health Care System", New England Journal of Medicine, 362, January 2010, p. 98-99; online at: http://www.nejm.org/doi/full/10.1056/NEJMp0910064 (accessed July 21, 2014)

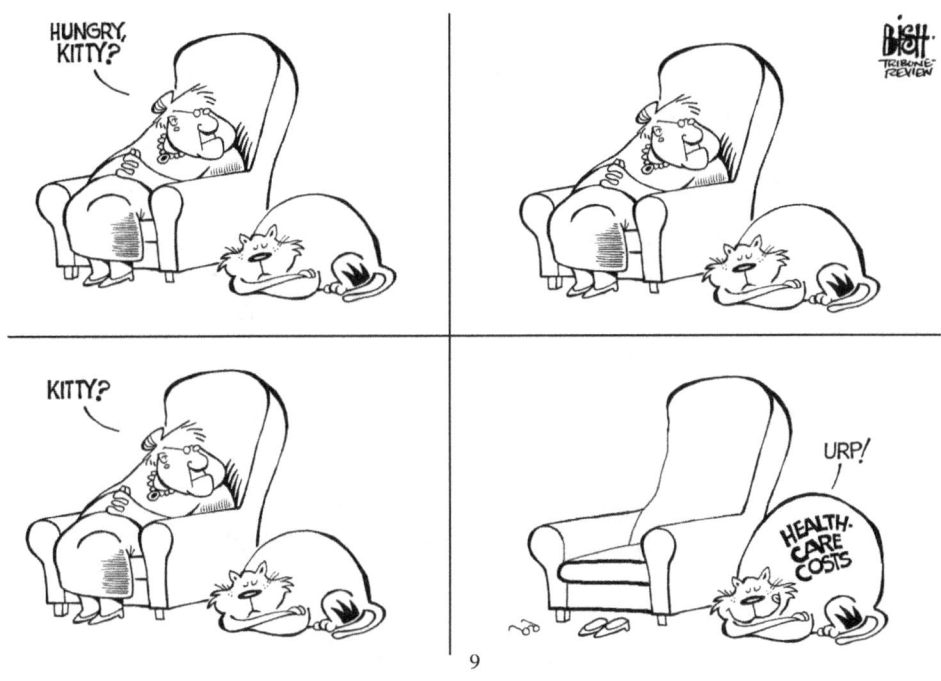

Health care is a vital service, not just some luxury. Health care is not merely a private matter for which the government should *butt-out*. The provision of health is not some optional, extra-curricular activity. *Health care is a must-have,* like police and fire protection or standard public education. Just as we have baselines for these critical, taxpayer supported services; we must have a baseline standard of health care service and access for all Americans.

---

[9] Bish cartoon, Healthcare Costs, Tribune Review; reprinted with permission from Political Cartoons.com

We can establish a baseline only after gaining a better understanding of the issues at play including:

- What are the most readily fixable problems in American health care?

- What cost-containment reforms actually promote the health and wellness of Americans?

- What is universal health care—really—and why is it such a hot button topic?

- What are the myths and realities of President Obama's Affordable Care Act?

- What can the average citizen do to help achieve meaningful reform that improves our health outcomes?

- What does " health care cost" really mean to you?

Stanford Emeritus Professor Fuchs, winner of the Distinguished Investigator and Distinguished Fellow Awards from the Association for Health Services Research, says, *"Major changes in health care policy usually occur because of something outside of health policy- large scale civil unrest, a depression. We cannot expect that change will be generated within a system. There is not enough desire for change, as opposed to desire on the part of many stakeholders not to change."*[10] In other words, health care consumers cannot expect health care

---

[10] Gina Kolkata, Knotty Challenges in Health Care Costs, New York Times, March 5, 2012,Sec. D p.6 ; online at: http://www.nytimes.com/2012/03/06/health/policy/an-interview-with-victor-fuchs-on-health-care-costs.html?module=Search&mabReward=relbia (accessed July 21, 2014)

industry insiders or our government to change an industry that benefits them unless *we* force that change. We cannot be change-makers without adequately understanding the issues, problems, and possible solutions. If America is to be healed we will have to heal ourselves and that healing starts with knowledge.

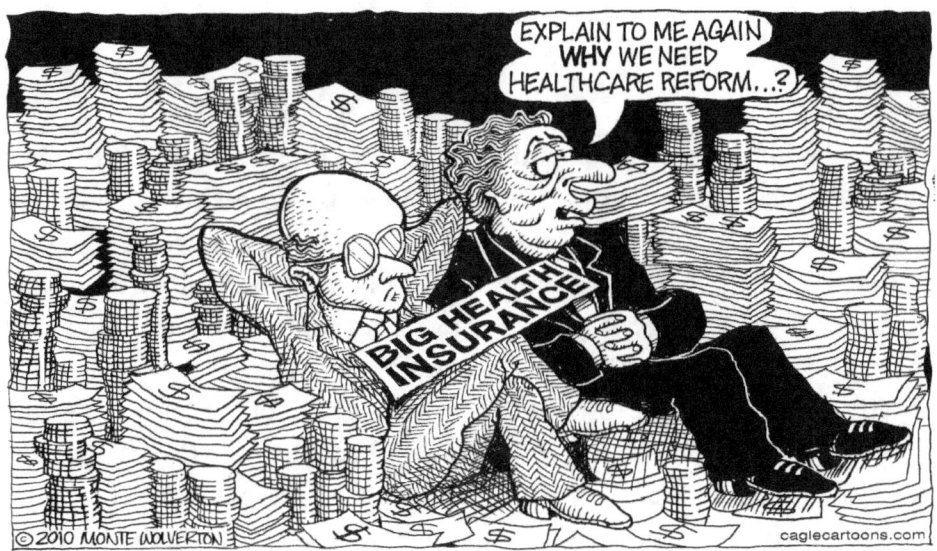

(Wolverton)[11]

---

[11] Monte Wolverton, Big Health Insurance; Permission to reprint this cartoon was granted by Political Cartoons.com

# Chapter 2

## *What's All this Talk about "Obamacare"*

Officially, the Patient Protection and Affordable Care Act (PPACA), which some health care reform opponents originally derided as "Obamacare", was signed into law by President Barack Obama on March 23, 2010.[12] (Obamacare, as a label, has since fallen into more neutral everyday usage, especially since the Supreme Court upheld the main provisions of the PPACA[13]). The PPACA passed the Senate by a strictly party line vote of 60-39, with all Democrats supporting and every Republican rejecting the bill.[14] The Patient Protection and Accountable Care Act passed the House of Representatives by a 219-212 vote, with all Republicans and 34 Democrats opposing the law.[15]

---

[12] Health and Human Services.gov, PPACA Healthcare Facts Timeline, March 23, 2010; online at: http://www.hhs.gov/healthcare/facts/timeline/index.html (accessed July 22, 2014). See also Sheryl Gay Stolberg and Robert Pear, Obama Signs Health Care Overhaul Bill, With a Flourish, New York Times, March 23, 2010; online at: http://www.nytimes.com/2010/03/24/health/policy/24health.html?_r=0 (accessed July 22, 2014).

[13] Adam Liptak, Supreme Court Upholds Health Care Law, 5-4 in a Victory for Obama, New York Times, June 23, 2012; online at: http://www.nytimes.com/2012/06/29/us/supreme-court-lets-health-law-largely-stand.html?pagewanted=all (accessed July 22, 2014)

[14] United States Congress Legislative Tracking, Bill 396, 111th Congress, December 2009; online at: https://www.govtrack.us/congress/votes/111-2009/s396 (accessed July 22, 2014)

[15] United States Congress Legislative Tracking, House Bill 165, 111th Congress, March 2010; online at: https://www.govtrack.us/congress/votes/111-2010/h165 (accessed July 22, 2014)

Since most of the significant and tangible aspects of the law did not take effect until 2014, both critics and supporters of the act are mainly guessing at what its full impact might be. Right or wrong, several of the issues the Affordable Care Act addresses have been agenda items for previous presidential platforms of both major political parties. Hence, the law actually reflects what many American people continue to say they need and desire.

In fact, the federal law actually resembles the Massachusetts health care reform law of 2006 enacted by then Republican Governor Mitt Romney.[16] The Massachusetts law was heralded by many on both sides of the political aisles as a model of sound reform before President Obama sought to replicate that measure, implementing its provisions in all fifty states. Hence, it has been interesting to watch members of Congress overly politicize this law for clearly personal and not societal gains.

Several allegations against the Affordable Care Act infer that it is a government takeover, which would establish *death panels*, impose severe cuts to Medicare benefits, and also financially cripple small businesses, have been debunked as myths by non-partisan political watchdog groups and several economists. Yet, the mythological criticisms keep coming.

The overall intent of the law is to give the average American citizen or small business owner more protection against the powerful, big businesses that currently control the health care system and to extend coverage to millions more Americans. Further, there are several provisions in the law that keep our money in the health system for the actual provision of health care and out of the private bank accounts of many corporations.

---

[16] The Commonwealth of Massachusetts Legislative site, 2006 Laws, Chapter 58; online at: https://malegislature.gov/Laws/SessionLaws/Acts/2006/Chapter58 (accessed July 22, 2014)

# Salient Facts and Key Phrases for the Patient Protection and Affordable Care Act

Information on the provisions of the Affordable Care Act was drawn from the official Health and Human Services site, which was updated as recently as July 16, 2014.[17]

**Pre-existing conditions:** Insurance companies will be prohibited from denying coverage based on pre-existing illnesses and chronic conditions.

**Age 26:** Health insurers will be required to provide coverage for dependent children up to age 26.

**$88,000:** New health insurance subsidies were provided to families of four making up to $88,000 annually, or, put another way, those earning wages that are 400 percent higher than the federal poverty level in 2010, which is indexed for inflation in future years.

**$695 or 2.5 percent, whichever is greater:** Starting in 2016, the fine will apply to individuals who fail to purchase health care insurance. For the poorest uninsured Americans, the fine would be waived. Additional exemptions apply as well and may be found on the official government site for the Affordable Care Act.

**Doughnut hole:** Under current law, Medicare stops covering drug costs after a plan has spent more than $2,830 per beneficiary/patient on prescription drugs. Medicare drug benefits resume after an individual's out-of-pocket expenses exceed $4,550. Called the

---

[17] U.S. Department of Health and Human Services, Key Features of the Affordable Care Act, posted September 20, 2012 and updated July 16, 2014l online at: http://www.hhs.gov/healthcare/facts/bystate/Making-a-Difference-National.html#PAGE (accessed July 22, 2014)

doughnut hole, it will be closed by 2020.[18] (Closing the Coverage Gap-Medicare Prescription Drugs, 2014)

**Summary of Who Pays for the Affordable Care Act**

**(Information on the tax and user fee contributions to pay for the Affordable Care Act were drawn from official government sources unless otherwise noted. )[19]**

**$27 billion:** Health care revenue to our government is derived from imposing annual fees on manufacturers and importers of branded drugs.[20]

**$60 billion:** Revenue coming from annual fees paid to our government by health insurance providers.[21]

**$20 billion:** Revenue paid to our government from 2.3% excise tax on manufacturers and importers of certain medical devices.[22]

**This is roughly $107 billion dollars and is money that these industries formerly distributed to their CEO's and stockholders**

---

[18] Centers for Medicare and Medicaid.gov, Closing the Coverage Gap, Medicare Prescription Drugs Are Becoming More Affordable, government publication 11493.pdf, , revised February 2014, http://www.medicare.gov/pubs/pdf/11493.pdf, (accessed July 22, 2014)

[19] Congressional Budget Office, Updated Estimates of the Insurance Coverage Provisions of the Affordable Care Act, Appendix B publication 45010, http://www.cbo.gov/sites/default/files/cbofiles/attachments/45010-breakout-AppendixB.pdf (accessed July 22, 2014)

[20] John E. McDonough, "Inside National Health Reform," 2011, University of California Press, p. 263

[21] Modern Health Care, IRS Creates Plan on Collecting Taxes to Pay for Affordable Care Act, Cranes Detroit.com, December 2, 2013, online at: http://www.crainsdetroit.com/article/20131202/NEWS/131209970/irs-creates-plan-on-collecting-taxes-to-pay-for-affordable-care-act# (accessed July 22, 2014)

[22] Christina Merhar, New Health Insurance Industry Taxes, Zane Benefits.com, January 16, 2014; online at: http://www.zanebenefits.com/blog/bid/273632/New-Health-Insurance-Industry-Taxes (accessed July 22, 2014)

**prior to Obamacare, which will now be used to pay for actual health care services.**

**$210.2 billion:** Revenue generated by a 3.8% Medicare surcharge on investment income from Medicare individuals making over $200,000 and Medicare couples making over $250,000.[23]

**2.35%:** Eventual special tax rate for high-income earners with those revenues earmarked for helping finance Medicare Part A.[24]

**50 employees:** Companies with more than fifty employees will be required to pay a fee of $2,000 per worker if the company does not provide coverage and any of that company's workers, as a result, receive federal health care subsidies. The first thirty workers would be subtracted from the payment calculation.[25] Both Wal-mart[26] and Disney[27] have already offered more benefits to their employees to avoid this penalty.

---

23
http://health.burgess.house.gov/uploadedfiles/one_page_on_unearned_medicare_tax.pdf

[24] Kathleen Rosenow, High-Income Individuals to Pay Higher Medicare Taxes Starting in 2013, Towers, Watson.com, September 2012; online at: http://www.towerswatson.com/en-US/Insights/Newsletters/Americas/insider/2012/high-income-individuals-to-pay-higher-medicare-taxes-starting-in-2013 (accessed July 22, 2014)

[25] The Patient Protection and Affordable Care Act, Public Law 111-148, 111th Congress, p. 111-148; online at: www.gpo.gov/fdsys/pkg/PLAW-111publ148/pdf/PLAW-111publ148.pdf, (accessed July 22 2014)

[26] Rick Unger, Wal-Mart Returning to Full-time Workers Obamacare Not Such a Job Killer After All, Forbes.com, September 25, 2013; online at: http://www.forbes.com/sites/rickungar/2013/09/25/wal-mart-returning-to-full-time-workers-obamacare-not-such-a-job-killer-after-all/ (accessed July 22, 2014)

[27] Jason Garcia, "Disney Offers Full-time Jobs to 427 Part-timers Who Meet Obamacare Threshold", Orlando Sentinel, October 2, 2013; online at: http://articles.orlandosentinel.com/2013-10-02/business/os-disney-offers-full-time-jobs-to-part-timers-20131002_1_walt-disney-world-part-timers-service-trades-council, (accessed July 22, 2014)

**$2.7 billion:** Revenue paid to government from 10% tax imposed on indoor tanning services.[28]

**$32 billion:** Revenue paid to government from 40% tax imposed on insurance companies offering "Cadillac" health plans valued at more than $10,200 for individuals and $27,500 for families annually. This provision does have a cost-of-living escalation clause.[29]

In addition to its financial implications there are socially humane measures in The Affordable Care Act as well.

    a. Ends insurance company power to cap the amount of health care a person can receive in his or her lifetime.

    b. Requires insurance companies to cover preventive services free of charge.

    c. Prevents insurance companies from charging women more money than men.

    d. Stops insurances companies from cancelling coverage when someone gets sick.

    e. Gives tax credits to small business owners so they can afford to offer their employees full health care.

---

[28] Christina Merhar, "New Health Insurance Industry Taxes", Zane Benefits.com, January 16, 2014. See also Erin Kim, "Obamacare's Tanning Tax Here To Stay", CNN Money, June 28, 2012; online at: http://money.cnn.com/2012/06/28/pf/taxes/tanning-tax/ (accessed July 22, 2014)

[29] Christina Merhar, "New Health Insurance Industry Taxes," Zane Benefits.com, January 16, 2014;online at: http://zanebenefits.com/blog/bid/273632/New-Health-Insurance-Industry-Taxes (accessed July 22, 2014). See also Blaine G. Sato, "THE VALUE OF HEALTH AND WEALTH:ECONOMIC THEORY, ADMINISTRATION, AND VALUATION METHODS FOR CAPPING THEEMPLOYER SPONSORED INSURANCE TAX EXEMPTION"' Harvard Education Journals, October 2013; online at: http://www3.law.harvard.edu/journals/jol/files/2013/10/Saito-Note.pdf (accessed July 22, 2014)

Still there are some bad things about The Affordable Care Act that leaves millions of Americans exposed.

a. It still does not guarantee universal health care.
b. The working poor will still have to pay fairly significant sums to have medical insurance.
c. Very little of the unregulated private and corporate expenses in American health care are addressed or curtailed.
d. Americans will still spend more on health care administration than any other country in the world.
e. Corporations and stock options still remain the driving force behind health care because the PPACA still operates under a for-profit construct.

Regardless of its flaws and inherent weaknesses, the PPACA remains a breakthrough piece of legislation that puts the building blocks in place to turn American health care in the right direction. With the PPACA in place and enforced, millions and millions of Americans from all socioeconomic backgrounds will have access to better and more affordable health care. Will it cost more? Initially, providing health insurance to most of the population may cost more money, but not for the reasons you might assume.

Resistance to change costs more. Private companies fighting the law or parts of the law in court will initially cost more. Americans being blatantly lied to and scared away from accepting the provisions of the law will cost us more. Politicians refusing to allow the law to take effect in their states and districts will cost us more. Lobbyists paying politicians millions to sabotage the law will cost us more. If we could look past the lies, stand our ground and come together as a people, I am confident that the Patient Protection and Affordable Care Act will live up to its real name and represent a turning point in American history that we all can be proud of.

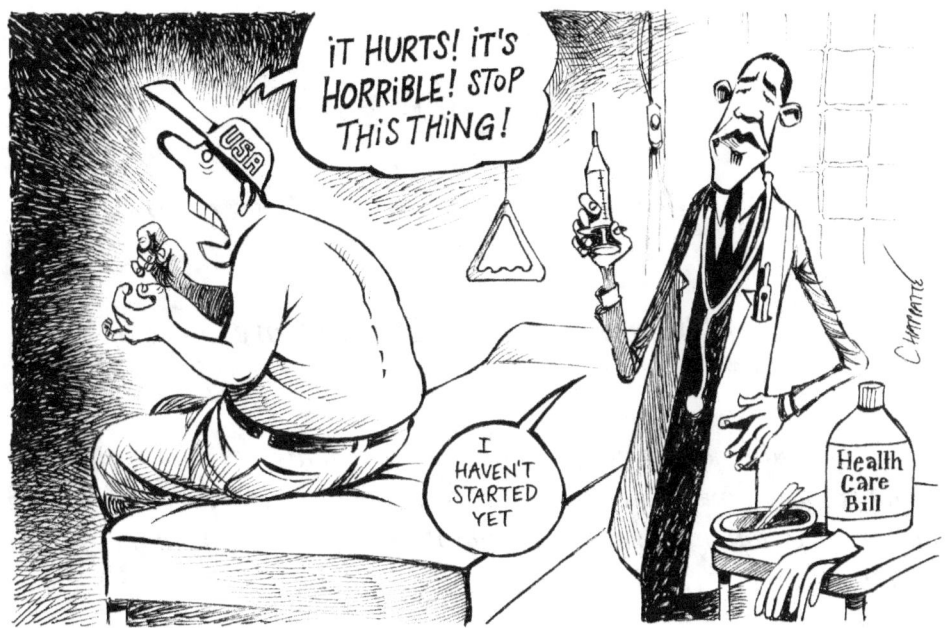

(Chapiatte)[30]

[30] Chapiatte, "Health Care Bill", has been reprinted with permission from Political Cartoons.com

# Chapter 3

## *Why Industrialized Nations (Except Ours)*

## *Choose Universal Health Care*

*"Health care is not just another commodity. It is not a gift to be rationed based on the ability to pay. It is time to make universal health insurance a national priority, so that the basic right to health care can finally become a reality for every American." U. S. Senator Edward Kennedy*[31]

Just recently, I treated a patient, Rod Mario. Mr. Mario is a fifty-four year old white male who owns a fairly successful flooring business with his cousin in northern New Jersey. Self-employed, Mr. Mario has an extremely limited medical insurance plan, which mainly covers injuries he or his employees might suffer on the job. You may wonder why he has such limited coverage. There are several reasons. Firstly, state law requires Mr. Mario have some form of injury coverage for his employees if he is to be in business. Secondly, the law does not require him to provide health insurance coverage to his employees, especially if he categorizes them as independent contractors.

---

[31]Senator Edward Kennedy, Quality Affordable Health Care for All Americans Kennedy, S. T. (2003). *Quality Affordable Health Care for All Americans.* National Institutes of Health. American Journal of Public Health., Journal of Public Health; online at: http://www.ncbi.nlm.nih.gov/pmc/articles/PMC1449947/ (accessed July 23, 2014)

Sadly, this nuance actually protects many small businesses because if Mr. Mario chose to purchase comprehensive health insurance independently he could easily pay $756 monthly for single employees and $1,352 monthly for family coverage, based on the latest information from the Kaiser Family Foundation Annual Survey of Employer Sponsored Health Benefits.[32] That is $9,072 and $16,351 a year respectively for each employee including himself for which he offered health insurance coverage. Even if he only pays for his employees individual insurance premium, that is nearly $10,000 yearly per employee. For a small business of only ten employees that means an expenditure of over $100,000 per year and this does not include the expensive injury liability coverage that is required by law[33] or dental coverage, eye coverage, business equipment, and salaries. Hence, without proper health coverage, Mr. Mario stayed at home for several days trying to tough out a nagging pain in his abdomen.

Unfortunately, that nagging pain turned out to be appendicitis and Mr. Mario's appendix perforated before he made it to the hospital. Even with all the technological innovations of the 21st Century, perforated appendicitis still carries a 5% mortality rate (5% or 5 out of 100 people afflicted will die) and 70% morbidity rate (70 out of 100 patients afflicted will experience medical complications). Fortunately, we were able to save Mr. Mario and discharged him after a five-day hospital admission. However, due to his lack of health insurance, Mr. Mario now has a $42,700 hospital bill to pay; it does not include the cost of his emergency room visit, post-operative visits, or his out-patient medications. **The United States of America is the ONLY industrialized country in the world where a taxpaying and working**

---

[32] Kaiser Family Foundation 2012-2013 Employer Sponsored Health Benefits Survey; online at: http://kaiserfamilyfoundation.files.wordpress.com/2013/08/8466-employer-health-benefits-2013_summary-of-findings2.pdf (accessed July 23, 2014)

[33] New Jersey Labor and Worker Development Department, Worker Compensation Requirements for Employers; online at: http://lwd.dol.state.nj.us/labor/wc/employer/require/insure_index.html, (accessed July 23, 2014)

**citizen like Mr. Mario has to live in financial fear of getting treatment for such an easily treatable ailment as appendicitis.** It is an embarrassment and shame that *we the people* should not tolerate any longer.

Let me be clear. Mr. Mario is not an outlier. On average, I see a patient like Mr. Mario at least once a month. In 2011, the memorable patient was Mr. Julio Camacho. Mr. Camacho was a fifty-one-year-old Latino male. He was an independent contractor and representative of the type of employees that Mr. Mario employed. Unlike Ms. Grayson whom I mentioned in the prologue, Mr. Camacho was a naturalized American citizen. Nevertheless, because of his insurance status, Mr. Camacho suffered for months with what he thought was indigestion. He finally was rushed to the emergency room during the winter holiday season with severe acute cholecystitis. We rushed him to surgery and removed his gangrenous gallbladder. Mr. Camacho then spent another nine days in the hospital fighting the infectious bacteria that his dead gallbladder had released into the rest of his body. Mr. Camacho told me his final hospital bill with ER charges was over $73,000.

Fortunately, both of these working Americans lived. However, there are many Americans who do not. For example, an obstetrical colleague of mine stopped taking ER calls after losing a twenty-four-year-old mom who went to the ER in full labor. The mom and baby died due to severe blood loss. This mother did not receive any pre-natal care. Why? Because she was convinced that despite advertising to the contrary, that her pre-natal care would cost her money that she and her husband just did not have. It would have been their second child and they wanted to save as much money as possible for the actual delivery of the baby. Of course, there are more medical nuances to this scenario. However, the major point is that all three of these tax-paying Americans made decisions that jeopardized their own health and safety solely because of fear of finances and costs. *Why are we allowing these tragedies to happen in one of the richest countries in world?*

A slew of political pundits, economists, lobbyists, policy advocates and policy-makers have described America's health care system as a quagmire. They say it's much too messy, muddled and bogged down to change it into what is conventionally termed as universal health care, a system granting access to anyone who wants and desires care and a method of delivering health care which is achieving good, measurable results around the world.

The disparaging barbs and dismissal of universal health care as unworkable in the United States are anything but true. A growing number of nations have proven otherwise. Australia, Belgium, Canada, France, Germany, Italy, Japan, South Korea, Switzerland, Taiwan, the United Kingdom, and several other leading industrialized and developing countries all have organized, implemented, and launched successful systems of universal health care. Most have done so within the last sixty years.

Though not perfect, these systems are delivering better outcomes than the United States. Far from an example of backwoods medicine, communist socialism, or any of the other disparaging names attached to universal health care by American detractors, such a system, in fact, is a marker of modern civilization. In 2014, the United States of America remains the only industrialized country that does not guarantee health coverage to every citizen regardless of income or employment status.

The following world map shows all the countries with forms of universal health care in shaded grey. Please note that the United States is the same color as less developed regions like India, Ethiopia, Pakistan, Uganda, Bolivia, Peru, and Mongolia. Worse yet, less wealthy countries like Chile, Uruguay, Taiwan, and even Sri Lanka have universal health care. This suggests that universal health care is achievable at low costs. To give you even more to consider, countries like India are providing quality health care at much lower costs than the United States, even when travel costs are factored in without a national healthcare system.

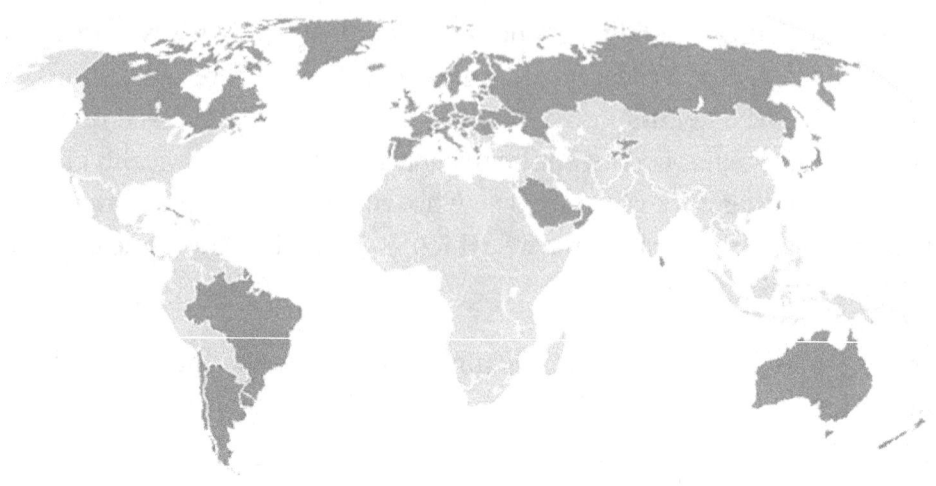

Choosing not to follow the global trend toward universal health care has neither been a smart investment nor good medicine for the United States. Though a global leader in myriad other arenas, our nation ranked last in the Commonwealth Fund's *Mirror, Mirror, On the Wall: How the Performance of the U.S. Health Care System Compares Internationally*[34], not only in 2010 but also in 2004, 2006 and 2007.[35] In the 2014 update of this survey, the United States ranked 46th out of all of the countries in the survey.[36] The U.S. trailed countries like Australia, Canada, Germany, New Zealand, the Netherlands, and the United Kingdom. The Netherlands, which switched to universal health

---

[34] The Commonwealth Fund's rankings are based on surveys of patients and physicians regarding various aspects of medical access, patient safety, coordination, efficiency, and equity. The surveys can be found on the Commonwealthfund.org web site.

[35] Karen Davis, Cathy Schoen, and Kristof Stremikas, "Mirror Mirror on the Wall: How the U.S. Healthy System Compares Internationally, 2010 Update; online at http://www.commonwealthfund.org/publications/fund-reports/2010/jun/mirror-mirror-update (accessed July 23, 2014)

[36] Karen Davis, Kristof Stremikas, David Squires, and Cathy Schoen, "Mirror Mirror on the Wall, 2014 Update: How the U.S. Health System Compares Internationally; online at: http://www.commonwealthfund.org/publications/fund-reports/2014/jun/mirror-mirror (accessed July 23, 2014)

care in 2006 and spends half of what the U.S. spends annually on health care, ranked No. 1 in health outcomes by 2010. The U.S. pays more money for these comparatively poorer health outcomes. The U.S. spent an average of $8,000 per person in 2009, exceeding per capita medical expenditures of 12 other leading, industrialized countries, according to a May 2012 study from the Commonwealth Fund.[37] Next up were Switzerland and Norway, spending $5,000 per person. [38]

Who can truly, credibly argue that the United States is unable to accomplish what other innovative nations are achieving through universal health care? The biggest challenge, of course, is deciding how to structure and operate a universal health care system to suit our American tastes and needs.

I believe universal health care is the best, fairest, most financially prudent approach. As we make our way towards a more equitable health system, there are prices, service delivery models, and performance to compare. "Comparative policy analysis" is what economists and policy experts call this process. And that leads us to four, relatively easy-to-understand, basic models of health care delivery: the Bismarck Model, Beveridge Model, National Health Insurance Model, and the Out-of-Pocket Model, which are listed in chart displayed at the end of this chapter. More detailed explanations on the different health system models from which to base national health care are found in the exhibits below.

---

[37] David Squires, Explaining High Health Care Spending in the United States, et, al, May 2012, p.2 ; online at:
http://www.commonwealthfund.org/~/media/Files/Publications/Issue%20Brief/2012/May/1595_Squires_explaining_high_hlt_care_spending_intl_brief.pdf (accessed July 23, 2014)

[38] David Squires, Explaining High Health Care Spending in the United States, et, al, May 2012, p.2 ; online at:
http://www.commonwealthfund.org/~/media/Files/Publications/Issue%20Brief/2012/May/1595_Squires_explaining_high_hlt_care_spending_intl_brief.pdf (accessed July 23, 2014)

## Bismarck Model

Founded in the 19th Century by Prussian Chancellor Otto Van Bismarck, the Bismark health care delivery model is actually similar to what exists for most working Americans today.[39] When Bismarck unified the Prussian Empire into Germany, he sought to garner both trust and power for his new government partly by creating private health insurance groups that employers and employees financed through payroll deductions. But unlike, say, Blue Cross and Blue Shield and other American insurers angling to turn a profit, Bismarck health insurer groups operate at-cost. They reinvest, or roll over, surplus revenue generated in Operating Year A into Operating Year B, which ensures a relatively steady flow of cash to spend on medical care. Further, these insurer groups must cover all people regardless of their employment status or ability to pay. Additionally, while German doctors and hospitals operate privately, they collect patient fees that are strictly set, controlled, and overseen by the government. Lastly, the government also strictly monitors the costs of medical supplies and pharmaceuticals. Belgium, Japan, Switzerland, and France also follow the Bismarck model.

## Beveridge Model.

Developed by British economist William Beveridge, the Beveridge Model is notably identified as a single-payer system.[40] Health care, like police protection and public schools, is financed by taxes paid to the government. Hospitals and clinics are usually government-operated, while doctors can choose to work privately or under auspices of the

---

[39] Physicians for a National Health Program.org, Health Systems-Four Basic Models; online at:
http://www.pnhp.org/single_payer_resources/health_care_systems_four_basic_models.php (accessed July 23, 2014)

[40] Physicians for a National Health Program.org, Health Systems-Four Basic Models; online at:
http://www.pnhp.org/single_payer_resources/health_care_systems_four_basic_models.php (accessed July 23, 2014)

government. Under the government-run, single-payer format, costs for services, payments to doctors and hospitals, available treatment options, and treatment outcomes all are more easily monitored and controlled.

Although Beveridge's native Great Britain is the most popular example of the Beveridge model, Cuba is probably the purest example of what Beveridge intended. The job of government, Beveridge contended, was to fight the "giant evils" of want, disease, ignorance, squalor, and idleness. To that end, as World War II raged, Beveridge collaborated with Ernest Bevin, then Britain's labor minister, to ensure that all Britons would have ready access to health care. Britain has since allowed the wealthy to pay out of their own pockets for services not rendered under its National Institute for Health and Clinical Excellence (NICE), while still maintaining their health care insurance coverage. Cuba, however, upholds the full ideals of Beveridge's brand of socialist medicine by giving the same options, same access and same health care financing to everyone. Other countries utilizing the Beveridge model include Finland, Denmark, Italy, Spain, and Norway.

**National Health Insurance Model**.

The national health insurance model, also known as the "Tommy Douglas model," is named for the Canadian politician who created Canada's first single-payer universal health system. This model of health care delivery is often described as a combination of Beveridge and Bismarck. It follows the Beveridge model's single-payer tenet and Bismarck's private insurer construct. The Tommy Douglas model was launched in Saskatchewan, the politician's home province, in 1962. Initially, doctors in the province resisted and went on strike. However, after quickly coming to terms on physician payment, the strike ended and the plan thrived. Amid much debate, the entire remainder of Canada adopted that model four years later. They called it "Medicare," the term the United States government borrowed when creating our own health care program for the aged in 1965. Canada's national system covers citizens under various insurance groups, while hospitals and doctors summarily are paid by one source. Canada's National Health Service is among the most prominent models of national health insurance in the world.

## Out-of-Pocket Model

The absence and opposite of universal health care, is the Out-of-Pocket model[41] and unfortunately, this is the most common health care delivery model in the world. In more than three-quarters of the world's approximately 200 countries, patients/consumers pay directly out-of-pocket for their health care or pay premiums in advance to a medical insurer for health care. Needless to say, such a system makes health care a luxury and not a right. It is a system unfairly weighted in favor of the rich. It exposes those with marginal incomes to the risk of going their entire lives without ever seeing a doctor or a dentist. In these countries, life expectancy is shorter, infant mortality is higher, dental disease is worse, and preventable disease is rampant. Further, most of these countries are underdeveloped and suffer from poor infrastructure or unstable democracies.

---

[41] Physicians for a National Health Program.org, Health Systems-Four Basic Models; online at:
http://www.pnhp.org/single_payer_resources/health_care_systems_four_basic_mo dels.php (accessed July 23, 2014)

| Models of Health Care | Pros | Cons | Where model exists | Average % of GDP that model accounts for: |
|---|---|---|---|---|
| Bismarck | Not for-profit insurers.<br><br>Insurers compete for patients.<br><br>Patient choice. | Patients pay up front for care.<br><br>Access to but nominal screening or preventive medicine. | Belgium, Japan, Germany, France | 11.2% |
| Beveridge | Health care is a right.<br><br>Patients are not billed for anything.<br><br>Patients choose their doctors.<br><br>Strong focus on preventive medicine. | Government chooses available services and medicines. | United Kingdom, Cuba, Italy, Spain, Norway, Denmark | 8.7% |
| National Health Insurance | Private doctors and hospitals.<br><br>No co-pays or deductibles.<br><br>Low-cost medications | Long Wait Times for Some Services<br><br>Comparatively limited access to specialists. | Canada, Taiwan, South Korea | 10.4% |
| Out-of-Pocket | High competition.<br><br>Market drives (and selectively restricts) available technology. | High costs.<br><br>Money dictates patient access. | USA, Many Third World countries | 16% |

Anguished details of people living in some of the poorest countries are beamed into our homes via the 6 o'clock news, YouTube, and other media. Their impoverished peoples plead for some recognition of their plight and, to ease that plight, they ask for our dollars. In my own small way, I have tried to help, traveling on medical missions of mercy to places in Africa and the Caribbean. I went to deliver free health care to those in need.

As a society, we are good at showing up during natural and manmade disasters. We empathize with those whose lives have been wrecked. We say, 'Oh, those poor people.' We pity them while either not recognizing or turning a blind eye to the friend, colleague, or neighbor here in America who suffers from medical neglect and sickness that are the result of not having adequate health care. It is a classic example of cognitive dissonance and disconnection, a warped psychology.

As we seek a healing for the people of this nation, we have to avoid being hoodwinked by health reform naysayers. We have to avoid being overwhelmed by the confusing bureaucracy of our current system, its artifice, and run-on menu of acronyms that encapsulate where we are now. *HMOs, PPOs, ACOs, IPAs, CDOs and IMGs ...* None of these are comprehensive systems of health care delivery. They are business models more than they are models for providing health care in the purest sense of what health care means. In the broad scheme of things, they were designed with a *profit* agenda not a *help* agenda with measurable, worthy goals for health outcomes that make the difference in human lives.

The leading dialogues in health care often focus on costs, waste, technology or medications. There is too little talk of lives nobly saved, natural therapies or disease prevention, such issues that when mentioned, often are couched in financial terms rather than purely moral ones.

# Chapter 4

## *What's Really Happening in American Health Care*

At the end of each broadcast of one of my favorite, childhood cartoons, GI JOE: *A Real American Hero*, I was always reminded to stay educated and informed because "Knowing is half the battle." I'd like to share some of what I know, as a physician, firsthand about the inner workings of our multilayered and complicated health care system, which is not transparent and easy to understand. Even worse, there are people and corporations who are counting on your fear and confusion to make billions of dollars while limiting your access to quality health care.

After reading this chapter you should have a basic understanding of the active agents in our current health care system and these are important facts for every American to understand. A proper background and fact-filled framework lets us move forward on real reform. Armed with enough know-how, we can be our wise health care consumers and advocate better on behalf of one another.

We must begin to read and get a working knowledge of health care that goes beyond that which our individual doctors and health insurance plans provide. From this informed view, we must push for a more simplified health care delivery process. Complex terminology, multi-level processes, ambiguous goals, and what-not have overburdened our health care system with administrative bureaucracy which make it hard for the layperson to navigate that system. Knowing how things work may not be half the battle for health care reform, but it is definitely where the battle begins.

As we try to unravel this tangled mess, let's imagine our present health care system as a field sport. Then, let's define the field of play and assign the players, referees, methods for scoring, and even include penalties for breaking rules. Let's toss in some commentators to summarize the contests, either from the sidelines or from deep within the center of the action.

**The Players:**

**1. Doctors**.  Physicians are among the most high-profile players in the game of health care. Indeed, at least since the 1960s, prime-time TV series featuring doctors have ranked in Nielsen's Top 10. Despite all the seeming celebrity, however, physicians are not the gatekeepers. They are not the primary powerbrokers. Doctors—to borrow from the entertainment industry—are the "talent." They deliver health care but, under the current system, rarely set, if you will, the sporting rules. Physicians wanting to move beyond the constraints of being the "talent" have returned to school, seeking other advanced degrees that hopefully will free them to participate in more than just the "clinical" aspects of health care.

**2. Hospitals, clinics, and federally qualified health centers.** These institutions are providing 70% of all advanced and primary health care; everything from emergency room triage to surgery, obstetrics, and intensive care. These health care facilities have contractual relationships with and receive funding from the government. Even so-called private hospitals generally are receiving some type of federal funding through Medicare, Tri-Care, and other government programs.

As their name suggests, federally qualified health centers (FQHCs) rely heavily on government aid to keep their doors open. Often, they provide primary health care in rural and low-income urban communities where limited or no health care is available without these specially funded nonprofit organizations.   In many rural areas, Federally Qualified Health Centers are the only source of health care providing checkups, baby deliveries, and minor surgery to poor and underinsured Americans.

**3. Payers.** The government and private corporations are the payers. Medicare for the elderly and Medicaid for the jobless and the poorest of the working poor are the programs most immediately identified as government-run and taxpayer-financed. Under the Patient Protection and Affordable Care Act (Obamacare), the self-employed or under-employed earning no more than 133% of the federal poverty level can now get Medicaid. Previously that group could earn no more than 100% of the federal poverty level. Nevertheless, the great tragedy is that millions of those eligible for Medicaid do not enroll, largely because they are not aware that they are eligible.   Other Medicaid eligible individuals, who are often low-wage workers are too ashamed to ask for help or subject themselves to the not uncommon humiliations meted out against needy applicants at the Medicaid office. One of the biggest problems in American poverty is that it is not fully recorded and documented by the federal government.

Medicare is supported entirely by our federal tax dollars and is a health care program for those age sixty-five and over, whose recipients laud the system. Medicare, in every conceivable way, is a single-payer system akin to those in Europe, Canada, and elsewhere, which flies in the face of American critics of health care reform initiatives as dangerous socialism and the antithesis to the American way of life. Medicaid costs are shared between state and federal governments with the management of Medicaid left up to each state governments. We are, after all, a nation of republics.

Private insurers are the last in this trifecta of payers. They function like any other business and the biggest health insurers are some of America's largest corporations, which generate billions of dollars of annual revenue and are publicly traded on Wall Street. **Four health insurers, UnitedHealth Group, Wellpoint, Humana and Aetna, were listed in top 100 of the 2012 Fortune 500 list. All of the CEO's of these four corporations personally made more than $20,000 a day in 2011**. For example, United Health Group's Stephen Hemsley earned $13.4 million a year or $36,438 a day and WellPoint's Angela Braly earned $13.3 million a year or $36,164 per day while Aetna's Mark Bertolini netted $10.6 million annually or $28,767 each day and finally, Humana's Michael McCallister earned a mere$ 7.3million or $20,000/day.[42]

These four individuals alone personally take home forty-four million dollars of insurance premium payers' money each year.[43] This, of course does not factor in the hefty salaries that are also paid to members of their executive teams. While there are several limitations and price schedules on what is paid to hospitals, laboratories, and clinicians for your health care, there is not one single limitation on what these health insurer executives can pay themselves. More importantly, there are wide discrepancies for executive compensation between hospitals and insurers. Often higher compensation does not jive with better performance. Some states, such as Washington, now require hospitals to disclose their executive compensation each year, as a part of an initiative to learn more about the cost drivers in hospital charges.[44]

---

[42] AFL-CIO, "Corporate Watch-Paywatch-CEO Pay and You; online at: http://www.aflcio.org/Corporate-Watch/Paywatch-Archive/CEO-Pay-and-You/CEO-Pay-by-Industry, (accessed July 23, 2014)

[43] Elisabeth Rosenthal, M.D.'s are Not Medicine's Top Earners, New York Times, May 18, 2014; online at: http://www.nytimes.com/2014/05/18/sunday-review/doctors-salaries-are-not-the-big-cost.html?action=click&contentCollection=U.S.&module=RelatedCoverage&region=Marginalia&pgtype=article&_r=0 (accessed July 23, 2014)

[44] National Conference of State Legislatures, 2014 Update of Health Transparency and Disclosure of Provider Payments: State Actions; online at: http://www.ncsl.org/research/health/transparency-and-disclosure-health-costs.aspxhttps://www.blogger.com/blogger.g?blogID=398291908231826 9632#edit

**4. Employers**. Unless you are a veteran, legally disabled, or qualify for the federal poverty level, you probably obtain your health insurance through your employer. If you're self-employed or under-employed you still have several options for health care coverage. (Most are usually flat-out unaffordable and, for many who investigate that market, extremely confusing.) The public exchanges that the Obama administration has been promoting are primarily meant to help the self-employed, under-employed, and small businesses get better health insurance for their money.

Nearly 60% of funds paid annually toward health care for about 175 million American workers come from employer contributions, which are subsidized, by federal tax deductions and exemptions. However, based on the annual Kaiser Foundation survey of health insurance plans, 80% of employers require their employees to contribute to the cost of their insurance in 2009. And in 2009, only 49% of U.S. employers offered health insurance to their employees.[45] Often this means the employee is paying the entire cost to add their spouse or children to the health plan. Since health care benefits can often eat up as much as 25% of an employer's payroll expenses, some small businesses really do struggle to pay health care benefits. It is hardly uncommon for them to drop the coverage altogether. Still, without employer contributions our current system would completely collapse. According to the 2013 Kaiser Foundation Insurance Survey, 57% of employers now offer health insurance to their employees, which reflect an increase in plan sponsorship, largely due to the Patient Protection

---

or/target=post;postID=1007181378988003266;onPublishedMenu=allposts;o, (accessed July 23, 2014)

[45]Winter, Roberta E., Unraveling U.S. Health Care-A Personal Guide, Rowman & Littlefield, July 2013, page 4;
 online at: http://www.amazon.com/Unraveling-U-S-Health-Care-Personal/dp/1442222972 (accessed July 24, 2014)

and Affordable Care Act mandates and incentives.[46] Though the penalties for not offering health insurance to employees do not start until 2015, businesses have decided to participate in exchanges and also to obtain health plans through associations and private means.

**5. Intermediate and/or acute care facilities.** Usually nursing homes or rehabilitation centers are paid the health insurance from their patients and supplemental payments out of the patients' own pockets. They provide clinical services and bill privately for them. If you ever watched the Suze Orman Show, you probably have heard of long term care insurance to help protect you if you ever in end up in one of these facilities. Medicaid and Medicare tend to only help pay for acute care; specifically, care that requires direct physician supervision. As the population of aging Baby Boomers continues to outpace that of younger Americans and orthopedic and other surgeries for that constituency become more commonplace, these agencies are assuming a more pivotal role in health care. Many Americans are making difficult financial and personal choices as they look for ways to provide safe, affordable, and comfortable living conditions for seniors who cannot live alone.

**6. Health care product suppliers.** Purveyors of wheelchairs, walkers, glucose machines, ambulance services, intestinal staplers, or mechanical heart valves, are medical equipment suppliers whom annually reap big, big bucks. These are usually private, unregulated companies charging whatever fees the health care market can bear. There are no limitations on the price tags or more importantly the profit margins of hernia meshes, pacemaker implants, or joint prostheses. In a similar fashion to companies that make athletic shoes and apparel (Nike

---

[46] Kaiser Family Foundation 2013 Employer Health Benefits Survey, August 20, 2013; online at: http://kff.org/report-section/2013-summary-of-findings/, (accessed July 23, 2014)

and Adidas), these companies are allowed to charge hospitals hundreds and thousands of dollars for products that they mass-produce at far cheaper costs.

**7. Pharmaceutical companies.** An astonishing factoid: **Americans buy 47% of all pharmaceuticals sold worldwide.** Atop that, prescription drug abuse in America has become such a problem that the federal Centers for Disease Control and Prevention cited in 2009, that for the first time ever, death from prescription drug related deaths surpassed deaths from motor vehicle accidents.[47]

Spending on prescription drugs in 2004 helped the world's Top 10 pharmaceutical companies generate more than $139 billion in sales in the US alone.[48] In 2011, the American pharmaceutical tally rose to $319 billion in sales with slightly more than 4 billion prescriptions filled. As Americans get older, more obese, more depressed, more anxious, and more sedentary, so does our dependency on Big Pharma.

The following chart outlines sales by major pharmaceutical companies in 2004. Note the percentage of sales in the U.S.A.

---

[47] Centers for Disease Control and Prevention, "Drug Poisoning Deaths in the United States- 1980-2008" Margaret Warner, P., Li Hui Chen, P., Diane M. Makuc, D. R., & and Arialdi M. Miniño, M. (20111). *Drug Poisoning Deaths in the United States-1980-2008.* U.S. Centers for Disease Control and Prevention. Centers for Disease Control and Prevention. http://www.cdc.gov/nchs/data/databriefs/db81.htm, (accessed July 23, 2014)

[48] Health Strategies Consulting, LLC, Follow the Pill-Understanding the U.S. Commercial Pharmaceutical Supply Chain, Kaiser Family Foundation, July 2005, Publication #7296; online at: http://www.avalerehealth.net/research/docs/Follow_the_Pill.pdf (accessed July 23, 2014)

| Company | Corporate headquarters | Annual revenue in millions of U.S. dollars | Total sales, USD | Percentage of sales to U.S. customers |
|---|---|---|---|---|
| Pfizer | United States | 46,133 | 52,516 | 87.85% |
| GlaxoSmithKline | United Kingdom | 31,434 | 37,324 | 84.22% |
| Johnson & Johnson | U.S. | 22,190 | 47,348 | 46.87% |
| Merck | U.S. | 21,494 | 22,939 | 93.70% |
| AstraZeneca | U.S. | 21,426 | 21,426 | 100.00% |
| Novartis | Switzerland | 18,497 | 28,247 | 65.48% |
| Sanofi-Aventis | France | 17,861 | 18,711 | 95.46% |
| Roche | Switzerland | 17,460 | 25,168 | 69.37% |
| Bristol-Myers Squibb | U.S. | 15,482 | 19,380 | 79.89% |
| Wyeth | U.S. | 13,964 | 17,358 | 80.45% |
| Abbott | U.S. | 13,600 | 19,680 | 69.11% |
| Eli Lilly | U.S. | 13,059 | 13,858 | 94.23% |
| Takeda | Japan | 8,648 | 10,046 | 86.09% |
| Schering-Plough | U.S. | 6,417 | 8,272 | 77.57% |
| Bayer | Germany | 5,458 | 37,013 | 14.75% |

*Source: Davidson, Larry and Greblov, Gennadiy. "The Pharmaceutical Industry in the Global Economy."*
49

[49] Larry Davidson and Gennadiy Greblov, "The Pharmaceutical Industry In The Global Economy", 2005, Indiana University Kelley School of Business, Table 1.1

**8. Patients.** Of course, our health care industry exists because people get injured and ill. While health care "consumer" rings, to some folks' ears, as an empowering term, it is bereft of the compassion and mercy that every patient deserves, especially those dealing with chronic, high-cost illness. Nevertheless, "consumer" does highlight that health care is, to a great extent, a supply-and-demand industry.

## Fields of Play:

**1. Doctor's office.** Despite all the focus on hospitals, the reality is that roughly 85% of health care delivery usually takes place in a physician's office. Aside from the local emergency room, it is the first stop for many patients. Usually, there are no operating rooms or fancy, high-tech machines, only a doctor peering into ears, noses, throats, and so forth to gauge health. The doctor-patient relationship has been the bedrock of American medicine and the primary source of whatever arguable prestige that physicians receive. People may not like medicine or hospitals, but there are very few people who do not profess love for their own doctors. Because they want to be well, many entrust their well-being to their doctors.

**2. Hospitals.** Though many doctor's offices are often on or near a hospital campus, those offices still differ functionally and financially from hospitals. State regulations usually require that a hospital be an institution that can provide certain emergency services 24 hours a day, seven days a week. In the American health care system, hospitals often are the last line between life and death (while doctor's offices and clinics tend to provide basic care to fairly stable patients).

**3. Emergency Medical Services.** These on-site, mobile triage teams handle acute or traumatic health events before a patient is actually transferred to hospital for follow-up care. In medicine, we refer to their work as the "golden hour." The resuscitative and stabilizing care given by EMS professionals has saved an untold number of lives.

Unfortunately, even as they save lives, EMS care is increasingly costlier. During the years when Americans were losing health care in droves, emergency rooms had become a sole source of care for many who lost health care coverage. But today, EMS teams are providing an ever-expanding, scope of services that save more lives each year. The presumptive hope is that the PPACA will limit loss of coverage and the dependence on emergency rooms or urgent care centers for basic medical care.

**4. Hospice.** Comparatively new to American health care, these end-of-life services are gaining ground in public knowledge and acceptance. They have become a convenient, more compassionate middle-ground care for the dying and their families who want this transition to take place in a non-hospital and non-home setting.

**5. Internet.** Despite the continuing lack of Internet service for the poorest Americans and those living in the most remote regions of the country notwithstanding, a mounting number of Americans are accessing health care advice and instruction using virtual tools with smart phone apps and the like. Americans are using the Internet to ferret out the best and worst hospitals, doctors, and medications.

As the costs of their deductibles, co-pays, and insurance premiums soar, patients are increasingly exploring home remedies and alternative therapies. Physicians, hospitals and insurers are also conducting more and more of their business via the Internet.

## Referees:

**1. Federal Government.** Although no single agency comprehensively monitors our mammoth health care system, the federal government wields extensive influence via two agencies: the Department of Health and Human Services (HHS) and the Center for Medicaid and Medicare Services (CMS). As the administrator for Medicare, CMS sets policies for payment, patient care, and patient safety that the entire industry generally follows. Why? Because virtually every hospital and health care agency in the country participates in Medicare. (Remember that Medicare is basically the same universal health care that certain entities ridicule as socialist entitlements.) Hence, CMS guidelines are the de facto standard for measuring performance, organization, and care delivery. If a doctor or hospital loses their Medicare enrollment, that's a very bad sign; insurers, drug companies, and durable medical supply people run for the hills. The de-enrolled doctors and hospitals often lose many contracts and fall into financial ruin.

The official federal agency responsible for overseeing our healthcare landscape is the federal Department of Health and Human Services, which sets policies and standards for clinical, administrative, and financial practices of our nation's health care industry. The HHS secretary is a member of the president's cabinet and the highest-ranking government official overseeing a health care industry mainly consisting of private businesses. Indeed, HHS has significant power and influence, though the power is displayed more in public policy and standards and not the actual governance of the many private corporations that exist in health care. Hence, Americans remain at the mercy of many for-profit private health care purveyors. *(Remember what I said about our out-of-pocket model.)*

**2. Private insurers.** At first glance, there are hundreds of health care insurance providers. **But really, only about ten huge and powerful insurance companies either control or directly administer more than 85% of the health insurance market.**[50] In many ways, these private, for-profit institutions—barely accountable to even the government, which nominally regulates them—are the true gatekeepers. Health insurers such as Cigna, United Health Group, WellPoint, Aetna and Humana are perennial Fortune 100 companies reaping in millions of dollars in pure profit yearly. Their deep-pocketed

---

[50] Winter, Roberta E, Unraveling U.S. Health Care-A Personal Guide, Rowman & Littlefield, 2013, p. 172

lobbyists have been hugely influential in Washington and among state legislatures. In many ways, they make the rules, determine who can play, and dictate what the score is. They almost always win.

If you want to know more, check out *Deadly Spin: An Insurance Company Insider Speaks Out on How Corporate PR is Killing Health Care and Deceiving Americans.* This 2010 tome, penned by former Fortune 500 insurance company (CIGNA) executive Wendell Potter, outlines some of what has gone awry. In addition the website, www.opensecrets.org lists in clear and specific tables all the money that our political leaders are taking from lobbyists from various industries.

**3. State Government.** As administrators of Medicaid, state governments hold a substantial stake in health care. Financed jointly by state and federal revenue, Medicaid provides care to more than fifty million of our country's poorest citizens.[51] From 2004 to 2011, national Medicaid enrollment rose from 41.1 million to 52.6 million people.[52] Designed to be our country's safety net for poor people, many state Medicaid programs have been criticized for stringent eligibility criteria, complex bureaucracy, and minimalist health care. Yet with nearly 30 states being managed by Republican governors who oppose President Obama, Medicaid and other health programs for the poor underperform due to lack of proper political and financial support. If emergency rooms serve as the main source of care for the poor, it is no surprise that 16 of the nation's 25 busiest emergency departments in 2011 were in Republican lead states.[53]

---

[51] InsuredKidsNow.gov, Medicaid, CMS, found online at:
http://www.insurekidsnow.gov/medicaid/ (accessed July 23, 2014)
[52] Laura Snyder and Robin Rudowitz, with Eileen Ellis and Dennis Robert Medicaid Enrollment, June 2011 Snap shot
http://kaiserfamilyfoundation.files.wordpress.com/2013/01/8050-05.pdf (accessed July 23, 2014)

[53] Modern Healthcare's "By the Numbers". December 23, 2013. Pg10.

**4. Accreditation agencies**. For all the intense focus on accreditation, few hospitals are likely to stay in business without that seal of approval and the accreditation process itself is voluntary. No independent accreditation agency can actually shut down even the most sub-par institutions. Still, accreditation is crucial, because insurers and medical suppliers tend to blacklist unaccredited institutions.

The Joint Commission (TJC) and the Accreditation Commission for Health Care (ACHC) are two prominent, non-governmental entities deciding which hospitals, clinics, medical schools, and health care facilities meet the established standards for quality care and education. A much longer roster of accrediting agencies monitors various other aspects of health care.

**5. Research and Policy Agencies.** The Federal Drug Administration (FDA), National Institutes of Health (NIH), and Centers for Disease Control and Prevention (CDC) are government sponsored agencies that fall under the jurisdiction of the HHS Secretary. These agencies heavily influence and monitor the public health and health care resources of the United States. Medications have to be approved by the FDA, the CDC creates protocols of screening and vaccinations to maintain the public health and the NIH supports and monitors medical research. In fact, when U.S. News & Worlds Reports does its yearly top hospital and medical school rankings, the amount of NIH funding a hospital or medical school receives is one of the top factors. Of course one should remember, that *NIH funding has nothing to do with how well medical students are being taught or the quality of care patients receive at these institutions.*

## Rules:

There are few rules set in stone. While the government provides some key oversight and monitors, it has allowed health care to operate under the market principles of supply, demand, and payment. As impressive as the scope of the NIH, FDA and CDC may sound, their limited means of actual enforcement is mind-boggling. Too many areas of our health care system are allowed to operate on an honor system. In addition, there are multiple agencies involved each with their own rules and agendas. There is no central office for which every health care policing entity directly reports to. Nevertheless, here are a few universal rules:

a. Health care is basically cash & carry. If you do not have a means of paying for it, you are infinitely unlikely to get any care that is not emergency care. **In addition, you can be billed, taken to collections, and have your credit score ruined if you do not eventually pay for your emergency care.**

b. Legally, hospitals cannot deny anyone emergency care. Doctors can refuse to provide care only in their private offices. Otherwise doctors must treat patients they see while covering a hospital's emergency room or clinic. Most doctors do not mind this. Instead they are frustrated that these same patients who received free care can sue them at anytime. In 1986, President Ronald Reagan signed the Emergency Medical Treatment Active Labor Act or EMTALA which banned hospitals from denying care. (Good intentions with some unfortunate consequences.)

c. Hospital and physician fees are actually already set by Medicare and private insurers. Hence all the media hype about hospitals over charging patients and their insurers is misleading half-truths. If a hospital or physician happens to see a patient from an insurance payer that they do not participate with, they can charge whatever they want. Some key things to remember here are that the payers often will pay no more than 80% of the bill and often will refuse to pay the entire bill. Does a hospital charging $17,000 for an emergency room visit mean anything if no one actually pays that bill? (This will be important later when we talk about "real costs of health care".)

d. Employers have to provide health care only to full-time employees. (Remember Mr. Camacho from chapter 1.)

    e.  Neither patients, doctors, or hospitals can appeal to a true independent arbitrator when they disagree with health insurer decisions.

    f.  Insurers now have to spend a certain percentage of revenue on direct healthcare costs or give the money back. In 2013, $500 million in insurance premium refunds were paid to policyholders, thanks to provisions from the Patient Protection and Affordable Care Act (Obamacare), requiring insurers to spend 80% of premium contributions on the provision of care.[54]

    g.  You cannot lose your healthcare just because you are sick, also a provision of Obamacare.

## Scoring Points:

When the endgame goals for these assorted players are, in fact, so disparate and conflicting, it can be hard to figure out which players are gaining ground. Nevertheless, there are ways to score points, with cost-containment being one of the biggest.

This whole idea of controlling health care cost fueled the once booming managed care industry, which dictates when, where, how, and from whom patients can receive care and precisely what doctors will get paid for providing various kinds of care. But twenty years into the managed care experiment, health care costs continue to soar. These troubling cost increases have pushed, over the last five years or so, disease prevention and better quality of care to the forefront of the cost-containment dialogue. The logic is that keeping people healthier in the first place will forestall expensive care later on.

Terms such as "evidence-based medicine", "quality control", or "value-based medicine" are concepts that place patient outcomes over patient

---

[54] Sy Mukherjee, "Insurers to Rebate Consumers 500 Million as a Result of Obamacare," Think Progress.org, June 21, 2014; online at: http://thinkprogress.org/health/2013/06/21/2194141/obamacare-big-insurers-overcharging/ (accessed July 23, 2014)

volume. Up until now, American medicine focused on volume and not outcomes. For example doctors, hospitals, pharmacies, etc. were usually paid based on the number of patients seen, number of surgeries performed, or number of pills dispensed. Volume drives the system and the costs. In this process, scoring points are based upon volume. Today, several agencies and groups including the U.S. government are pushing the linkage of payments to clinical outcomes and not just volume.

In the very near future, hospitals and clinicians will either get paid bonuses or have penalties levied against them based on the health quality outcomes of the healthcare that they give. This has already happened. The Accountable Care Act has already had two years of operation and has paid bonuses to organizations that are participating in the Accountable Care Program. For instance, hospitals are now being penalized if patients with certain diseases are re-admitted to a hospital within 30 days of their discharge. To learn more about paradigms of quality care or value-based care, check out the Agency for Healthcare Research and Quality (AHRQ), the National Committee for Quality Assurance (NCQA), or look up medical homes. Interestingly this concept of "outcomes health care" that will control *costs* has been the pet project of various Democratic and Republican presidents for at least twenty-five years.

However, the major problem is no one knows what our actual health system costs are. Even more importantly the term costs means something different to every player on the field. Of course, the group that suffers the most from the complex confusion is you, the consumer/patient. In her book *Who Killed Health Care,* Harvard Professor of Business Administration Regina Herzlinger argues that the biggest problem in American health care in not just cost but lack of a universal definition for what constitutes our health system costs. [55]

---

[55] Regina Herzlinger, "Who Killed Health Care-America's $2 Trillion Dollar Medical Problem and the Consumer Driven Cure", McGraw Hill, 2007; online at: http://www.amazon.com/Who-Killed-Health-Care-Consumer-Driven/dp/0071487808 (accessed July 23, 2014)

Indeed when someone is discussing cost in health care they could be referring any one of the following:

- Health insurer payments/spending
- Insurer premiums
- Federal government health care spending
- Hospital spending
- Hospital pricing or charges
- Employer health care payment/spending
- Medical goods and supplies

Hence, when Joe Patient goes to a hospital or doctor he has absolutely no idea what he is exactly paying for or why he is paying it; even car buying isn't that bad. The EOB (Explanation of Benefits) on insurance company statements or patient medical bills rarely give useful financial information. EOB's are just one of example of the lack of real transparency which have fueled blame gaming, price inflation, fraud, and monopoly. Even hospitals do not always know what their expenses are. Hospitals do not pay the same price for the exact same medical and surgical supplies. I think one of the fairest ways to assess the various health care players as generators of costs would be to start with their profit margins. I am certain that most Americans would be shocked if they were able to see the true profit margins of their health insurers, hospitals, pharmaceutical companies, physician practices, or our federal government. In addition, what are the costs and expenditures of any financial relationships that federally sponsored agencies such as the National Institute of Health, Centers for Disease Control, Federal Drug Administration and National Cancer Institute may have with private health care companies? These are health care related agencies that are supported by your tax dollars but none of their workers are directly accountable to the public.

Although these agencies report to Congress, in many ways they remain unaccountable to the public. For example, when the FDA approves cancer drugs like Sanofi's Zaltrap or more recently Merck's Keytruda through an expedited process that is 60 days or less, is it all based on clinical incentive? Both Zaltrap and Keytruda cost more than $11,000 a month to administrate and can easily cost more than $100,000 per patient for a complete treatment course. The expedited review process the FDA uses is barely 60 days. Merck was recently allowed to skip several common phases of clinical testing to market Keytruda.[56] Who decides to rush such expensive and extremely profitable drugs to market? Indeed cancer doctors like Memorial Sloan Kettering's Leonard Saltz and University of Chicago's Richard Larson have begun to question the costs of these rapidly approved drugs.[57] Yes, the FDA, NIH and CDC are public agencies but a horrific quagmire of political bureaucracy and lobbying negates any true accountability. What are the real profit margins of your local hospital or your local Blue Cross? Who is really operating under financial duress, our local hospitals or local health insurers?

## Commentators:

**1. Surgeon general**. Honorifically known as America's Doctor, the Surgeon General provides the broad public with information and resources on healthy living. Unlike the federal secretary of Health and Human Services, the surgeon general, whose office is within HHS, only makes recommendations and does not enforce policy. Sadly this office has remained vacant for most of President Obama's tenure due to Republican led Senate rejection of all his nominees.

**2. Media.** The multi-billion dollar health care micro-economy deservedly gets plenty of media attention. It is a necessary focus, though I am quite concerned that the American popular media are not providing enough fair and balanced information. Depending on what you read or where you tune in, you may be getting only part of the story. The news coverage has become entertainment and way too

---

[56] Andrew Pollack, F.D.A. Allows First Use of a Novel Cancer Drug. New York Times, September, 5, 2014, Sec. B pg.1.

[57] Stephen S. Hall, "The Cost of Living" New York, October, 28, 2013: 25-29.

politicized, relying on the fast sound bite rather than rolling out explanatory journalism that gives Americans all of the facts and, based on solid journalistic standards. Consequently, when Americans attempt to make decisions on health care reform, there are far too many opinions and not enough objective facts in the popular American media.

To be sure, much of the less commercialized popular media, such as The Economist, The Nation, or longtime investigative and explanatory veteran journalists such as Public Broadcasting's Bill Moyer, provide a more impartial conveyance of the facts. It is important, as information consumers, to include them in your sources. If we are to make informed decisions we must also seek accurate knowledge from which to draw conclusions.

**3. Policy Experts and Advocates**. Because health care reform has been a hot-potato political issue for at least thirty years, a veritable universe of individuals and organizations proffering frequently colliding facts and opinion has grown up around the reform debate. Although they rarely consist of practicing physicians, they usually serve one of five aspects:

(1) Advisors presenting non-partisan, unbiased, empirical information about reform

(2) Pawns of partisan agenda peddlers often supported with paychecks from lobbyists for health care titans who do not want change

(3) Media Sources—whether reasoned or ridiculous—for news reporters on the health care beat

(4) Think tanks whose leaders realize the desperate need for change and are actively researching various reform models

(5) Politicians who view health care and the health care debate as a path to the limelight and a long legislative career.

One can find a lot of policy expert articles on the Huffington Post, the Kaiser Family Foundation, and the Commonwealth Fund websites.

| GROUP | EXAMPLES | FUNCTION |
|---|---|---|
| **Players** | Doctors, hospitals and clinics, payers, employers, intermediate and acute care facilities, health care products suppliers, pharmaceutical companies, patients. | Participate in and determine health care delivery and access. |
| **Fields of Play** | Doctors' offices, hospitals, EMS Services, hospice, Internet. | Actual venues where health care is delivered. |
| **Referees** | Government (CMS & HHS), private insurers. | Agencies and corporations that decide how health care should be delivered and governed. |
| **Rules** | Very little that is universal, clear or objective (too many chefs and not enough waiters) | Laws and instructions governing the practice and business of health care. |
| **Points** | Agency for Healthcare Research & Quality (AHRQ), National Committee for Quality Assurance (NCQA), The Joint Commission. | The accepted goals of health care currently: quality outcomes and cost-containment |
| **Commentators** | Surgeon General, media, policy experts and advocates. | People who and agencies that heavily influence public opinion on health care. |

On the surface, doctors and the patients for whom they are sworn to give care consume much of the spotlight. However, in the actual debate over how to remake American health care, they are in many ways, the odd-person-out. Money remains the key driver and determinant.

Physicians, hospitals, insurers, pharmaceuticals firms, even medical schools, nursing schools, physician assistant schools, and so forth are focused on how to turn a profit. That is not to say that every player operates with the wrong motive. Indeed, there are many operating nobly, with healing and good health in mind. Health care remains one of the biggest sources of charity in the nation. Yearly, doctors, hospitals, and clinics give away millions of dollars in free health care. I am certain that they would give away more if they did not have their own bills to pay.

Although I am obviously biased, please note that physicians are the only party in health care who are required to take an oath of fairness, ethics, and decency. Moreover, clinicians are the only players in the game who can also lose their ability to practice medicine over issues of fairness, ethics or decency. Have you ever asked yourself, "Why is it so difficult to sue an insurance company or a pharmaceutical company?"

Please do not misunderstand me, I am a capitalist and proud of it. I like competition and the idea of open markets. But the cleric in me firmly believes that money making, of any sort, must have a conscience. It must have some moral undergirding and foundation. When money becomes the primary aim in health care, it causes suffering among innocents, among those who are the economically most disadvantaged and, during this lingering Great Recession, among the hordes of formerly middle-class, uninsured and under-insured families being forced to forego a necessary visit to the doctor in order to put food on the table.

In a land of plenty, it is unconscionable that anyone has to make these kinds of choices.

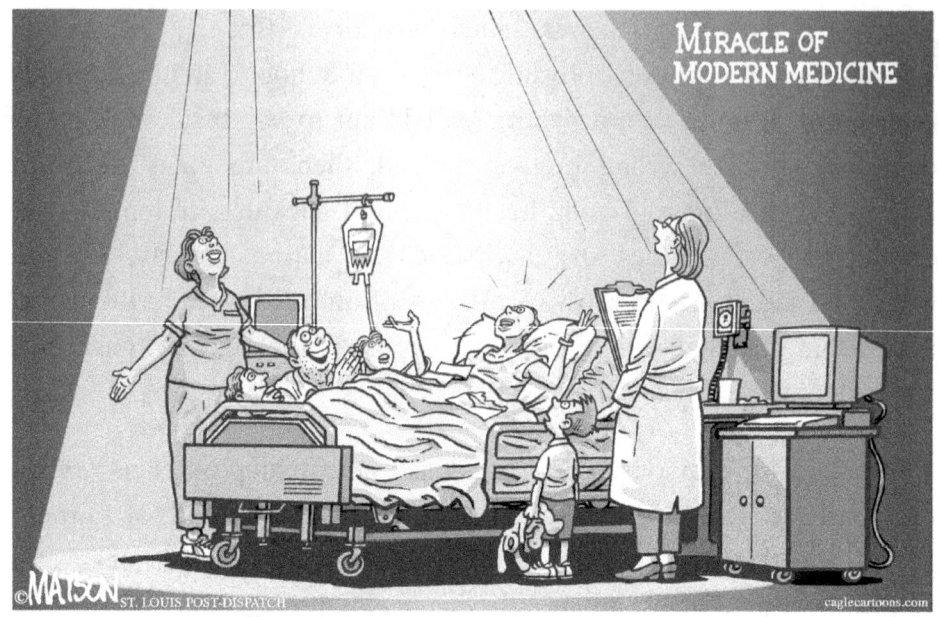

"OUR INSURANCE COMPANY WILL PAY!"

(Matson)[58]

I believe we want to win on the health care reform front. I believe that the *want* is real.

The last four presidential administrations were attuned to our often desperate, collective desire to change and improve the health care system. Those presidents have known that much was at stake.

In turn, we, the people, have wanted lowered costs, better service, and easier use interface for our health system. An October 2009, Associate Press-GFK Roper Media poll revealed that although only 40% of those surveyed supported the PPACA, 62% of those polled in that same survey, said they wanted President Obama and Congress, especially the

---

[58] Matson, "Our Insurance Company Will Pay," St. Louis Dispatch, reprinted with permission from Political Cartoons.com

Republicans, to pass a major health care reform law.[59] Other polls suggesting that there is some groundswell of opposition to health care reform fail to distinguish those who are fundamentally against change from those who say the present changes do not go far enough. Without additional reforms, we will never have a system that extends access to care, across the board, and yields a healthier America.

---

[59] GFK Roper Media, "AP-GFK Health Care Reform Survey-2009"; online at: http://surveys.ap.org/data%5CGfK%5CAP-GfK%20Poll%20Final%20Healthcare%20Topline%2020100609.pdf (accessed July 23, 2014)

# Chapter 5

## *Why Doctors Are Angry and Why You Should Be Angry, Too*

### Doctors are often blamed for what is wrong in health care

What is the major problem in American Health care? Costs! Who are the biggest drivers of costs? Physicians. Physician order tests, prescribe medications, perform procedures, all of which get portrayed as negative events with cause for suspicion. This practice is neatly summed up and euphemized in the term utilization. Every hospital, large medical practice, and health insurer has some sort of utilization review process. This whole process primarily exists to teach physicians how not be wasteful and not generate needless medical costs. This ideology confuses physicians because physicians are taught to investigate, to diagnosis, to treat, to help, or to do something. Utilization exists to make sure that the least amount of care within legal limits is given. Utilization reviews often put physicians on the defensive by demanding explanation of all your medical treatments. At its core, utilization is a great thing for American medicine. Unfortunately, utilization does not address the ever increasing cost of administration and oversight in medicine. Nor does it address the unregulated costs of durable medical goods, pharmaceuticals, or medical supplies. These are extreme costs in health care that clinicians have no control over or for which they are frequently held accountable.

## They have little say in medical finances

For all their prestige and fame, physicians have comparatively little input in how health care dollars are actually spent. Hence, being frequently blamed for wasting health care dollars only adds insult to the injury of being left out of the health care expenditure conversation. Now many health care policy advocates and insurer lobbyists will say this is not true. On the contrary, it is. The few physicians who have meaningful input on health care spending occupy non-clinical administrative positions. This may seem like a minimal issue but consider that hospitals and lawmakers routinely make sweeping health care decisions without any dialogue with the actual clinicians who will be affected by their decision. Whole departments or clinical units will be opened or closed with little to no dialogue with the actual clinicians involved.

Moreover, the American Medical Association (AMA) is one of the most popular and oldest medical groups in the U.S. Yet the AMA has absolutely no official seat at the tables where national health care finances and utilization practices are discussed. Neither the Centers for Medicare, Department of Health and Human Services, nor Congress have an official AMA liaison. This lack of political respect and power is a key reason why in recent years AMA membership have fallen to less than 25% of practicing physicians in the U.S.

## Their medical expertise is routinely questioned

Physicians undergo the longest and arguably most difficult training of any profession by far. American physicians spend a minimum of 7 years in post-graduate study with the average being around 9 years. Compare that to 3 years for lawyers, 2 years for stock brokers and bankers, and 4 to 5 years for other doctoral degrees. Yet physician judgment, skill set, and overall competence are routinely second-guessed and called into question. This occurs despite physicians consistently being tested, retested, certified, and recertified in order to maintain their practicing privileges. No other profession including lawyers and bankers are held to such high standards of competency.

On one hand, this makes sense because physicians literally are responsible for other people's lives. On the other hand, it is baffling that, at times, physicians have to answer to non-clinical people with only legal or financial backgrounds. Lawyers do not answer to non-lawyers regarding legal competence and financers do not answer to non-financiers regarding financial competence. Yet physicians are often questioned by non-physicians regarding their practice methods. Amazingly health insurers, pharmaceuticals, and medical suppliers rarely answer to anyone. Think about it. How often do you hear of a company in one those three fields get penalized for anything by anyone. Although the Centers for Medicare and Medicaid admit that less than 2% of physicians commit fraud, we routinely hear stories and media exposes about physician and hospital fraud.

In addition, despite of all of their training, physicians are frequently encouraged, if not outright forced, to follow universal algorithms and paradigms in a "one size fits all" motif. Although this mindset aids in upholding a standard of care and quality, it also downplays the diversity of humanity and the myriad of ways diseases affect us. There are indeed patients who do not fit in algorithms.

## Doctors are financially struggling

Contrary to popular belief, a significant percentage of working physicians are facing extreme financial hardship and struggle to pay their bills. This fact sharply contrasts with the public expectation that after all their hard work and training, all physicians live comfortably without financial worry.

**In July 2012, the Quantia Physician Wellbeing Index (Quantia Inc., 2012) stated that: 26% of primary care physician reported poor financial health, 43% of physicians reported trouble covering the costs of their practice, and 18% of employed physicians reported salary reductions in the past two years.**[60] In addition, an April 2013, CNN-Money website article by Parija Kavilanz, reported that the American Bankruptcy Institute had noticed an increase in physicians filing for bankruptcy for causes not related to having lost a malpractice suit.[61]

When I attended medical school in the early 1990s, we were told do not worry about the money (referring to our med school loans), because for good doctors practicing good medicine, the money will take care of itself. Unfortunately, nearly twenty years later, nothing could be further from the truth. For most physicians, the money is not taking care of itself. These financial worries have led to increased physician burn out, cynicism, and bitterness. In a survey of 13,600 physicians done by the Physician's Foundation, 57.9% of physicians said that they would not recommend a career in medicine to their children and a whopping 84.2% felt that field of medicine was in decline.[62]

---

[60] Quantia Inc, Physician Wellbeing Index, findings posted July 31, 2012; online at: http://www.quantia-inc.com/news-blog/press-releases/struggling-primary-care-physicians-could-undermine-affordable-care-act/ (accessed July 23, 2014)

[61] Parija Kavilanz, Small Business Physicians Driven to Bankruptcy, CNN-Money, April 8 2013; online at: http://money.cnn.com/2013/04/08/smallbusiness/doctors-bankruptcy/ (accessed July 23, 2014)

[62] Merritt Hawkins Biennial Survey of American Physicians for the Physicians Foundation.org, September 2012;  online at:

# WHY AMERICANS (YOU) SHOULD BE ANGRY

## You are being denied care

One of the most embarrassing aspects of our society is how physically and mentally sick Americans are. We have the best technology in the world. Yet many Americans are blatantly denied access to care or miss out on decent care simply because of financial reasons. Very few of our health care resources are being over utilized. Instead they're being restricted and privatized like a luxury commodity. Since when did democracy mean unequal access to health or health care? If accused of a crime, you are guaranteed free access to legal counsel without any co-pays or expectation that you will pay for any of it. Yet somehow, when it comes to your health there is an expectation to pay for some of it. Moreover, if you whine about paying for your health care, you run the risk of being called a lazy freeloader. How does it make sense to make legal protection absolutely free while charging for health protection?

## You are being denied your basic Constitutional right

The preamble to the US Constitution reads as follows, "We the People of the United States, in Order to form a more perfect Union, establish Justice, insure domestic Tranquility, provide for the common defence, promote the general Welfare, and secure the Blessings of Liberty to ourselves and our Posterity, do ordain and establish this Constitution for the United States of America". Note that the words justice, tranquility, welfare, blessing and liberty are all preceded by action verbs proclaiming them as a basic right and priority. Still, two hundred years later, people are routinely denied the tranquility and welfare of

---

http://www.physiciansfoundation.org/uploads/default/Physicians_Foundation_2012 _Biennial_Survey.pdf (accessed July 23, 2014)

good health based largely on their economic status. Moreover, many of those same individuals, including people like me, who support their right to care, are now being called a socialist or communist if you expect universal healthcare. Yet universal health care is clearly consistent with the public policies promoted in the opening words of our Constitution. Even the 4$^{th}$ Amendment of the Constitution affirms the right for you to be secure in your own personhood. How is that possible if you are not guaranteed health care?

## You are being lied to

For more than forty years, Americans have been told that the basic right to being healthy costs too much. Every presidential administration since Lyndon Johnson has looked for some way to control health care costs. Meanwhile health care and health insurance has remained one of the most profitable industries over that same time period. While millions of Americans have suffered and died waiting for treatment, several individuals have amassed private fortunes. Money that could have been used to treat your family is instead being used to line the pockets of a select few. To add insult to injury, money is taken from your hard-earned paycheck only for you to be later told that you and your children are not sick enough to use it.

Finally, you are given outlandish numbers for health care costs such as $559.3 billion for Medicare and $896.3 billion by private insurers. What you are not told is that more than 30% of these expenditures are administrative costs.[63] Administrative costs include expenses such as salaries, marketing, utilization review, or lobbying. Yes, these costs can include the money spent on denying your health care treatment.

---

[63] Steffie Woolhandler, M.D., M.P.H., Terry Campbell, M.H.A. and David U. Himmelstein, M.D., Cost of Health Care Administration in the United States and Canada, New England Journal of Medicine,2003: 349:768-75: online at: http://www.pnhp.org/publications/nejmadmin.pdf (accessed July 23, 2014)

## You are being robbed

Working Americans via their employers, pay approximately $650 billion a year in insurance premiums. In addition, the government reportedly paid $882 billion of your tax dollars in 2011 on Medicare alone. Together that is $1.5 trillion of your money spent each year on health care. This does not include federal and state monies spent on Medicaid. Interestingly the U.S. Census estimated that total 2012 population was approximately 313 million. Generous estimates suggest that barely 250 million American have health care coverage and that at least 40 million have no health care coverage at all. Further still, even if you have insurance, you have to pay co-pays and deductibles for large portions of your care. Where is your money going? Why do you not know where your money is going? Why do you not receive detailed reports of how much of your health insurance premium is actually spent on you? Why is it hard for you to see transparent reports on what your doctor or hospital charged and what they were actually paid for your care? Why are you kept in the dark about the actual costs of your x-rays, blood test, or medications? What other industry is allowed to charge you so much based on so little information?

## Your health insurance coverage is a joke
## (assuming you're lucky enough to actually have insurance)

The health insurance lobby has done a wonderful job of presenting your health insurance as an undeserved entitlement. However, the average health insurance policy by no means covers everything. Mental health treatment, dental care, long-term care, physical therapy, vision care, and disability support are just some of the things that are left out of typical health insurance policies. In spite of all the hoopla about cost and utilization, health insurance usually only helps those of us already in good to moderate health. If you are unlucky enough to have a real medical issue that requires surgery, chemotherapy, or hospitalization large portions of the costs routinely get passed on to you. Costs such as anesthesia, pathology, or in-hospital consultations are frequent culprits. Your insurer can claim that none of these entities participate with them and pass on 80% of the costs directly to you; regardless of how much money you have been paying in yearly premiums. In fact, prior to the Patient Protection and Affordable Care Act (Obamacare) your insurer could change your specific benefit package without any fear of reprisal or charges of discrimination.

# Chapter 6

## *What We Can Do*

*Rationed care. Skyrocketing costs. Death mills.* Those are some of the inflammatory labels, lies, and mischaracterizations stoking fears about health care reform. They are part of what have stopped us in our tracks and kept average citizens from meaningful discussion and action on the issue.

But as we separate fact from fiction, we can get on with the reforms. So, here's the deal: Lobbyists for entrenched, reform-resistant players in the field of health care are busy feeding politicians their version of the story. Lobbyists argue their reasons for why the health care bosses need to keep making money. The politicians—some of them, anyhow—heed the lobbyists. Lobbyists are buying the politicians' votes.

Some voters end up regurgitating what the lobbyists and the un-reform-minded politicians erroneously spout. And for reasons more partisan than practical, some of the very Americans for whom the current health care construct is not working repeat what their favorite politicians spew. Unknowingly, these Americans are working against their own self-interests.

What is true is this: Almost every industry linked to health care has had an extremely lucrative run for at least the last forty years. Over fifty years, only national defense spending has been higher than that of health care.

## So where are the health care dollars? And what are they accomplishing—or not?

In 2011 alone, employers paid $552.8 billion—yes, billion, with a "b"—in premiums to health insurance companies, while total spending for all private health plans was 822.3 billion in 2010. This represents an increase in excess of 130% since 2000.[64] Compare that increase to a 42% wage increase for employees over the same time period. Remember what I said in Chapter 1, about healthcare costs crippling the American economy. The costs of health insurance premiums are literally putting companies out of business and/or keeping salaries frozen. Obamacare has provisions that require both health insurers and pharmaceuticals to pay more taxes back into the system. We, the people, just have to make sure that those tax costs do not get secretly passed on to us.

It is impossible to trace precisely where health insurers and pharmaceutical firms spend their money. It is hard to pinpoint executive salaries, stock dividends paid, and what is actually being spent providing health care to health consumers. These companies are not required to report, in simple, clear formats, what they do with money they're making from their customers. However, there are provisions in the PPACA (Obamacare) that will change much of that, as cited in Chapter 2.

In addition, although privately owned pharmaceutical companies have much of their research underwritten with government-allocated tax

---

[64] Centers for Medicare & Medicaid Services, "National Health Expenditure Projections 2010-2020", 2010; online at: http://www.cms.gov/Research-Statistics-Data-and-Systems/Statistics-Trends-and-Reports/NationalHealthExpendData/downloads/proj2010.pdf (accessed July 25, 2014)

dollars, so do all of the nation's top medical schools and hospitals. There is no valid reason that their financial records should remain a mystery. Although the Sunshine Act[65] (Medicaid) now requires physicians and hospitals to report any monies or gifts received from private health care related companies, such as pharmaceutical or medical device manufacturing corporations, this is only a small step into the light. Moreover, it does not address the gross financial mis-management that is taking place in many hospitals and medical institutions. For instance why would a state regulatory authority allow executives who are sent to temporarily oversee the restructuring of a hospital which is in financial duress, to receive $700 an hour in compensation? More importantly why aren't there any regulations preventing such payments. A hospital that could not afford to pay medical supplies cannot afford to pay someone who does not treat patients $700 an hour.[66]

To repeat my mantra: The battle to save our health care system begins with each of us getting up to speed on the available information and demanding greater transparency and disclosure of what is now hidden. (Remember, knowing is where the battle begins!!)

Hence, Step 1 is nudging our lawmakers to make all financial records and holdings of every sector of the health care industry publicly available. Here are some other cost sectors that warrant being monitored and adjusted:

**Administration.** In spite of all the talk about ballooning costs in health care, it is rarely mentioned that America spends more money on health care administration than any other country in the world. Please note health care administration is completely separate from health care delivery. In short, these are not expenses that clinicians and patients generate. These are costs generated by third parties who tell clinicians

---

[65] http://www.cms.gov/Regulations-and-Guidance/Legislation/National-Physician-Payment-Transparency-Program/index.html
[66] Crain's Health Pulse, "The Price of Leadership", July, 08, 2014, Pg. 1.

and patients what to do. **In 2011, 14% of health care expenditures in the U.S. were related to administrative costs to an estimated $361 billion.**[67]

Who are these people doing the managing? A behind-the-scenes cast that include, but isn't limited to chief executive officers, chief financial officers, chief utilization officers, chief quality officers, chief medical officers, and clinical chairpersons. And these are just the people who work in a hospital. On the other side of the fence, the insurers have a full phalanx of personnel determining which patients are eligible for which services and the level of payment to be recouped for dispensing those services. Unfortunately, administration is only one area of inflated expenses. Here are five others:

**1. Physician expenses.** Again the U.S. leads the world in a negative aspect of health care. American physicians pay more money for their education and to continue practicing than the rest of their international peers. Student loan repayment, malpractice insurance payments and office overhead make staying in business a real challenge for doctors.

Currently, the average American physician graduates from medical school with $150,612 to $176,675 in student loan debt. This generally translates into approximately $1,800 to $2,300 a month, including interest, in loan repayments for several years. [68]

Malpractice coverage can range anywhere from $6,000 to $95,000 a year, depending upon a doctor's location and specialty.[69] A 2011

---

[67] Physicians Foundation Whitepaper-Drivers of Health Care Costs, November 1, 2012; online at:
http://www.physiciansfoundation.org/uploads/default/Drivers_of_Health_Care_Costs_-_November_2012.pdf (accessed July 24, 2014)

[68] 2011 Medical Student Loan Debt, Association of American Medical Colleges, October 2011; online at:
(https://www.aamc.org/download/309346/data/11debtfactcard.pdf), (accessed July 24, 2014)

[69] Physicians Foundation Whitepaper-Drivers of Health Care Costs, November 1, 2012; online at:

survey by Profiles, which bills itself as a resource for physician recruiters and recruitment, found that 21 of 51 specialists earned about $300,000 a year.[70] Imagine having to siphon off $80,000 of that just for malpractice insurance. And we have not even begun to discuss the operational and overhead costs of being in private practice.

**2. Employer expenses.** Typically, health insurers increase their premiums whether or not their costs of covering a given employer's employees have actually jumped. The federal government should intervene by mandating stricter and clearer guidelines about when premiums can rise and by how much.

Certain states have similar provisions to control insurance premium hikes. Some judiciously exercise those controls; others do not. The whole process should be far less piecemeal. Moreover, if we continue with a for-profit model, employers should at least be allowed their fair share of health insurers' profits, which employers ostensibly are underwriting.

**3. Prescription costs.** Of all U.S. pharmaceutical companies ranked in the Top 10 for earnings in 2008, the highest earning drug company was Pfizer with $44.4 billion in posted earnings in the previous year. The net profit of this powerhouse was $8.1 billion.[71] The lowest gross revenue reported was by Wyeth Laboratories, which grossed $17

---

http://www.physiciansfoundation.org/uploads/default/Drivers_of_Health_Care_Cos ts_-_November_2012.pdf (accessed July 24, 2014)
[70] 2011-2012 Physician Salary Survey, Profiles Database.com, published 2013; online at: http://www.profilesdatabase.com/resources/2011-2012-physician-salary-survey (accessed July 24, 2014)
[71] http://www.pfizer.com/files/annualreport/2007/financial/financial2007.pdf

billion. [72] Their financial statements reported a net profit of $4.6 billion for fiscal year 2007. [73]

## Top 20 Pharmaceutical Companies

| | | |
|---|---|---|
| 01 | Pfizer | $44,424 |
| 02 | GlaxoSmithKline | $38,501 |
| 03 | Sanofi-Aventis | $38,452 |
| 04 | AstraZeneca | $28,713 |
| 05 | Merck | $26,532 |
| 06 | Novartis | $25,477 |
| 07 | Johnson & Johnson | $24,866 |
| 08 | Roche | $21,998 |
| 09 | Eli Lilly & Co. | $17,638 |
| 10 | Wyeth | $17,179 |
| 11 | Bristol-Myers Squibb | $15,622 |
| 12 | Abbott Laboratories | $14,632 |
| 13 | Schering-Plough | $12,773 |
| 14 | Bayer Schering | $12,294 |
| 15 | Boehringer Ingelheim | $11,103 |
| 16 | Takeda | $10,626 |
| 17 | Astellas* | $8,530 |
| 18 | Daiichi-Sankyo* | $7,382 |
| 19 | Eisai* | $6,250 |
| 20 | UCB Group* | $4,370 |

*Based on 2007 pharma revenues.*

*Note: In all Top Company profiles, dollar amounts are in millions. -*
*See more at:* http://www.contractpharma.com/issues/2008-07/view_features/2008-top-20-pharmaceutical-companies-report/#sthash.hWXXHx1S.dpuf

---

[72] 2008 Top 20 Pharmaceutical Companies, Contractpharmac.com, July 18, 2008; online at: http://www.contractpharma.com/issues/2008- 07/view_features/2008-top-20-pharmaceutical-companies-report/, (accessed July 24, 2014)
[73] http://library.corporate-ir.net/library/78/781/78193/items/283760/Wyeth_FR_07_lo.pdf

While pharmaceutical companies often claim that research-and-development costs are driving up the costs of new medication, they spend just 13.4% of their revenues on R&D, according to researchers at York University. In 2008, U.S. pharmaceutical firms spent an average of 24.4% of sales revenue on marketing and promotions.[74] Basically, pharmaceuticals spend twice the amount of money advertising their products as they do creating them. This phenomena stems from a precedent setting law which allows pharmaceutical companies to advertise directly to consumers. The US is one of only two countries which allow this practice that increases demand for products which may not otherwise be requested by consumers. Essentially we are paying higher prices for our prescription drugs because of advertising.

**The United States of America remains the only G-7 country in the world that does not regulate what pharmaceutical firms can charge for their drugs, which is particularly troublesome for the elderly.** When drugs costs became inconceivably high, the federal government did craft Medicare Part D to cushion users of that prescription plan from the blow of those unchecked rising costs. The supplemental Medicare Part D helps pay for the drugs and keeps seniors supplied with what they need.

**4. Medical durable goods.** Medical supplies such as glucose machines, wheelchairs, and orthotics are part of an unregulated market. Therefore, Americans and, where applicable, their insurance companies, are paying through the nose for those supplies.

**5. Technology** For a few years, I sat on a New York City Department of Health task force investigating why women of color were less likely than white women to get a mammogram to screen for breast cancer. A surprising finding was that all the mammogram centers in the city were being used at 70% to 80% of their actual capacity. So, there were more

---

[74] Gina Kolata, Knotty Challenges In Health Care Costs, The New York Times, March 5, 2012 ; online at: http://www.nytimes.com/2012/03/06/health/policy/an-interview-with-victor-fuchs-on-health-care-costs.html?_r=0; (accessed July 24, 2014)

than enough resources. The question, then, was what issues prevented people from fully accessing available care? Why were there more machines than seemingly necessary?

I am not advocating rationing or restricting care in some draconian way. Indeed, mammography is a necessary life-saving technology. However, there are several medical services in American health care that are not nearly as necessary as their inventors or paid physician spokespeople would suggest. What I am advocating are crystalline guidelines on where and how high-end equipment is deployed. A national, neutral board should be established, assuring that the numbers of tertiary services (cardiovascular, cancer or orthopedic) and equipment in a region match its population and health care demographics, not the local hospital's or physician practice's marketing plan.

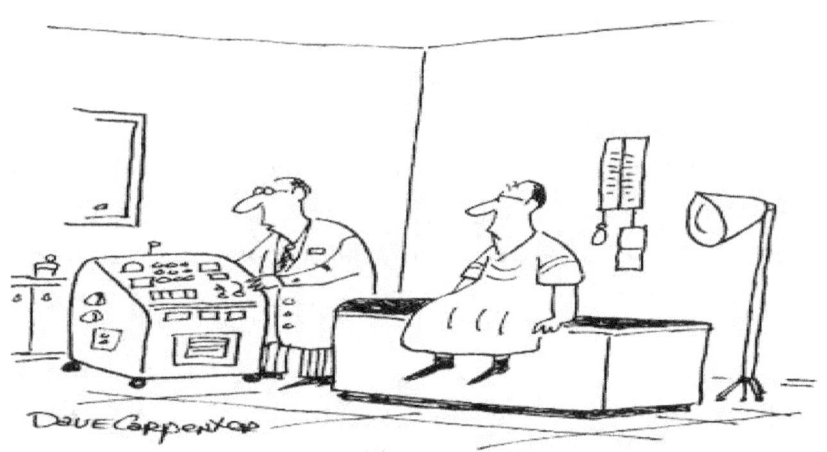

"First we're going to run some tests to help pay off the machine."

That is one aspect of our ongoing technological advancement to address, and the other is how competition for *"consumers,"* rather than patients, tends to force hospitals and physician groups to offer the newest technology even when that technology is still relatively unproven. That leads to too many MRI machines, Da Vinci robots, PET scans, dialysis centers, and even motorized wheelchairs and all are paid for by sometimes needlessly pumping up the number of patients who use those services and that fancy equipment. Stanford Professor Emeritus Fuchs calculated that, as one example, the U.S. has 4.2 times as many MRI scanners as Canada, our neighbor to the north whose universal health care system spends less money and gets better health outcomes.[75]

We have reviewed things that we should reduce or better control as part of reform. More efficient use of technology is one practical means of cutting costs. I believe properly implementing the following measures would not only reduce costs, but also improve patient outcomes.

**1. Universalized Electronic Medical Records (EMR) and Smart Cards.** As part of what now is a major push toward electronic medical record-keeping, the federal government has been offering substantial bonuses to hospitals and physicians who make that transition fast and early. The hope and presumption are that EMRs will reduce the number of medical errors, duplication of services, and improper screenings for illness, all of which drive up costs and medical complications. Well, except for this one small detail, EMRs might really live up to the hype and their touted purpose: There is no mandate that EMR systems have the built-in, automatic, easy capacity to link and communicate with each other.

Once again, capitalist competition in the health care market and financial profit won out over good clinical practice. Thus, if Hospital A has a different EMR system than Hospital B, just one zip code away, patients shuttling between hospitals still remain at risk for medical error, duplication of services, and interrupted continuity of care.

---

[75] Gina Kolata, Knotty Challenges In Health Care Costs, The New York Times, March 5, 2012 ; online at: http://www.nytimes.com/2012/03/06/health/policy/an-interview-with-victor-fuchs-on-health-care-costs.html?_r=0; (accessed July 24, 2014)

EMR innovators definitely should make money. But, as a collective, they should be in sync with each other, across all applications and platforms, even if it means uploading otherwise proprietary data to a central database.

Smart cards are another innovation. In an ideal world, they also would coexist with universal EMR communication systems. In France, for example, citizens have a card encrypted with all of the insurance information and medical encounters "Carte Vitale", regardless of which doctor or hospital previously provided care. Carte Vitale readers are plugged into every French doctor's office and every health care center. Thanks to this small tool, physicians and hospitals can easily track patients' history of care. They are currently testing a method of providing full clinical information and results on the cards. **Imagine going to a new doctor and handing them a smart card that will have the results of every blood test, vaccination, or x-ray that you ever had in your entire life.**

Making a secure national database of healthcare information for clinicians to access is easier than it sounds. Already every physician has a unique National Provider Identifier (NPI) number that's registered with the federal government. This number could be used to access and monitor all physician activity in the database. Further there is a organization called Health Level Seven International (HL-7) that has created a framework for the comprehensive integration and sharing of electronic health record information and it is called Open Systems Interconnection.[76] Furthermore, the five largest electronic health record system vendors (Epic Systems, Allscripts, eClinicalWorks, NextGen Healthcare and GE Healthcare) currently control fifty-five percent of the US market.[77] Linking just five software companies could change the entire face of the costs and efficiency of American Healthcare.

---

[76] http://www.hl7.org/implement/standards/product_section.cfm?section=4
[77] Modern Healthcare's "By the Numbers", December 13, 2013:37.

**2. Preventive Medicine**. Sadly, preventive medicine still exists as a kind of alternative therapy in the American psyche, rather than a daily health focus and habit. The reasons why are baffling. The merits of preventive care are proven. In 1950, for example, British researchers Richard Doll and A. Bradford Hill verified that cigarette smoke causes lung cancer. In 1973, U.S. President Richard Nixon declared war on cancer by urging better screening and identification of risk factors. Some Americans have gotten the hint that their personal efforts to stay healthy do make a difference. Declining tobacco use, for example, has been attended by declining deaths from lung cancer among men since 1990.

### That's a bit of the good news. There's also the bad news.

Across socioeconomic status, substantial numbers of Americans tend to look to health care as the antidote after we have done the self-damage. Specifically, we tend to seek clinical help only when we think something is wrong. Our current health care system does not adequately promote or reward preparatory or preventive interaction with clinicians. Some described this as transactional care versus value-based care. We Americans tend to visit our doctor's once we have succumbed to disease that could have been thwarted with good nutrition, exercise, and avoidance of unhealthy excesses of alcohol, cigarettes, abuses of illegal and prescription drugs. Many of us who are insured do not take advantage of obvious, accessible forms of other prevention. Despite the availability of screenings for several types of cancer, which are often offered for free at community clinics, no more than 80% of people at risk for cancers are screened.

I could go on and on … If costs are to be significantly reined in, then American patients and American physicians must put a lifestyle of prevention front and center. Diet, exercise, and meditation would certainly be part of that equation.

**3. Universal Health Care.** I absolutely could not help but come back to this point.

Increasingly we are a nation of part-time workers. The Bureau of Labor Statistics counted a record-breaking trend of 34.8 million of them in 2012.[78] Of course these workers do not qualify for health care benefits; a fact that world's largest retailer WalMart has capitalized on. Even those of us lucky enough to have full-time jobs continue to see our menu of benefits shrink and grow more expensive at the same time.

Assuring tax-funded universal health coverage for *every* citizen, regardless of employment status, offers several potential benefits:

- Larger pools of payers.

- More equal distribution of high-disease, high-risk insured people across health insurers.

- All employers contribute to a national fund.

- Better continuity of care and preventive medicine.

- Decreased paperwork and administrative expenses as coverage remains more constant and centralized.

---

[78] United States Census Bureau, Labor Force Survey Press Release, 2012-103; online at: http://www.census.gov.ph/old/data/pressrelease/2012/lf1204tx.html, (accessed July 24, 2014)

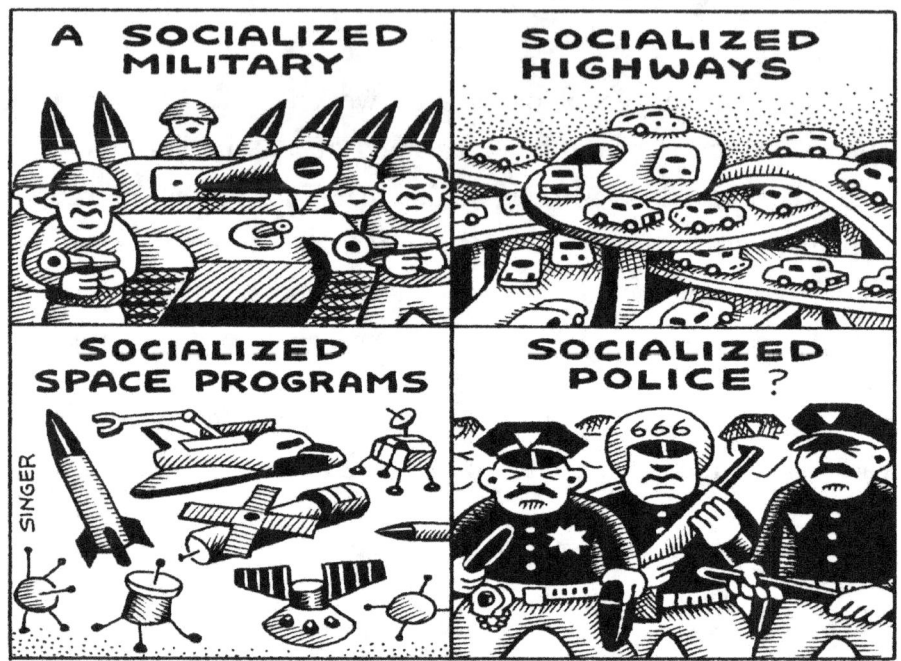

[79] (Singer)

**4. Remove the "for-profit" motive**. This final task is also probably the most important. This concept is so crucial that a large commercial insurer, Nationwide, mentions it in their national marketing campaign: *"We put members first, because we do not have shareholders."* **If a commercial home and auto insurer can admit that having shareholders might compromise its integrity for its customers, why do we feel that health care is any different?** Wherever profit is the penultimate aspiration, there can be no equality of access amongst individuals needing finite health care resources.

---

[79] Andy Singer, "No Exit"; reprinted with permission from Political Cartoons.com

The notion of curbing profit in certain sectors of our health care industry so that no one is on the margins of health care is a distasteful, unimaginable idea to some. Nevertheless, it has become clear to me that profit cannot be the driving goal or benchmark of a health care industry that is going to survive and thrive over the long haul.

Indeed, health care should be a right for all peoples, not a dispensable luxury for an increasingly moneyed few. The ultimate goal should be coverage and proper care for all, not fat stock options for the few happy shareholders. Market forces and enriched shareholders should not unduly influence the kind of care we make available to anyone, everywhere. This ideal of equality of care supersedes all others.

Using the latest Congressional Budget Report, 31 million people are projected to have insurance coverage due to the Affordable Care Act. **Still, between 26 million and 27 million are expected to remain uninsured until and unless another sweeping reform comes to pass.**[80]

Great Britain and Canada overhauled their systems, granting health care to all, shortly after World War II. More recently, Taiwan and South Korea adopted a similar system of universal coverage. So, what is the "what next" for our great country? How will we, the people, resolve this urgent matter? To whom are we beholding? What changes will we demand that move America into a more thoroughly modern kind of medicine?

---

[80] Congressional Budget Office, Updated Report on the Effects of the Insurance Provisions of the Affordable Care Act, April 2014;  online at: http://www.cbo.gov/sites/default/files/cbofiles/attachments/45231-ACA_Estimates.pdf (accessed July 24, 2014)

*Seven changes that will create real health care reform and equality:*

| | |
|---|---|
| **Full Transparency** | How can we adequately discuss money if we don't have all the facts? |
| **Restructured and pared expenses** | Several of our health care expenses are arbitrarily inflated. The term "cost" has to have a more consistent definition. |
| **Regionalized tertiary care and utilization** | We really have more technology than we require. Don't be fooled. New is not always better. |
| **EMRs and smart cards** | Use the digital age to connect and unite our health care system as opposed to increasing fragmentation. |
| **Preventive medicine** | Move from "find-it/fix-it" transactional care to "avoid-it/prepare for it" value-based care. |
| **Universal health care** | Anything else is simply immoral. |
| **Remove profit motive** | Human lives should not be counted in terms of "medical loss ratios." |

# Chapter 7

## *What You Can Do*

*"Never doubt that a small group of thoughtful, committed citizens can change the world. Indeed, it is the only thing that ever has."*

—Margaret Mead, anthropologist, co-drafter of the Episcopal Common Book of Prayer (Bowman-Kruhm, 2003)

Christianity started with one leader and 12 disciples.

- Judaism started with three patriarchs.

- Fifty-six men signed the U.S. Declaration of Independence.

- There were five original officers of the Southern Christian Leadership Conference, the central force of the Civil Rights Movement, including the Rev. Dr. Martin Luther King, Jr.

Those iconic leaders and followers banded together and changed the world. Though they were a mere handful of ordinary, bold, convicted folks, they influenced government officials, titans of industry, and the people next door.

As it relates to health care reform, ours would not be the first generation to persuade political and business leaders to create much needed change. After all, we pay their salaries, whether by voting them into office or purchasing the myriad products they peddle. For the health reform-minded, whether individual activists or members of advocacy organizations, it is a matter of demanding that our public and private officials supply what we want in the way of health care. What follows are descriptions of various groups that many of us fall into and a partial prescription of what we can do, via those groups or on our own, to pursue real, true reform.

**1. Faith-based groups.** At least 200 million Americans regularly participate in religious activity. That is more people than the nearly 167 million people the 2010 U.S. Census counted across California, Florida, Georgia, Illinois, Michigan, New York, North Carolina, Ohio, Pennsylvania and Texas combined. There are more than enough God-focused Americans to fulfill what I see as a moral, ethical, and religious mandate to make sure no one in our human family is refused his or her God-given right to quality health care. If faith-based organizations alone mobilized their memberships—through petitions drives and resolutions, on picket lines and in legislative corridors—just imagine how persuasive that would be.

**2. Social organizations.** From the Lions, Kiwanis, and Rotary Clubs to fraternities, sororities, secret societies, and professional organizations to our friends on Facebook, Twitter, LinkedIn, Tumblr, or Instagram, we have drummed up enough to collective clout and contacts to be real change-makers. It amazes me how many professional organizations have remained on the sidelines of reform. Indeed commentary and public service ads on smoking, obesity, abortion, or alcohol abuse all have their place but where are the public statements on corporate cash and carry in health care. Where are the statements from the American Heart Association, American Cancer Association, American College of Surgeons or American College of Pediatrics? Where are the ethical manifestos from the Catholic Church, the Baptists, the Methodists, or Episcopalians? Americans are literally dying from lack of health care reform and several key organizations have remained silent on the issue of reform.

That kind of en masse organizing to guarantee full health care coverage to every American would be a community service project and cultural shift of epic proportions. In fact, it might be the defining work of our generation. Our generation could be the generation that saved American healthcare!

**3. Teens, college students and young adults.** The young are more likely, given their relatively good health, to feel a sense of invincibility, if not a near immortality. Yet, these are some of their potential realities:

- Work prospects of young Americans have diminished during the Great Recession. Given the forecast of a long and, so far, tenuous, economic recovery, many of our adolescents are biding their time by staying in college and earning advanced degrees. They need more viable health care options than the campus health center.

- Adolescents and young adults frequently hold part-time and/or contractual jobs that do not offer health care benefits. It is not unlikely that many will still be in those kinds of jobs after age 26 when the Affordable Care Act no longer lets them remain on their parents' insurance. However, they can obtain subsidized insurance through the various insurance exchanges (assuming they remain intact). They will then be able to pursue health insurance through the government exchange. Often, the lack of healthy living and proper preventive care in our twenties sets people up for suffering in our fifties and onward, which impacts the urgency of health education and surveillance in the early years.

We cannot risk leaving youth and young adults out of this equation. They have been on the frontlines of many a social and political movement in this country. They have often been willing to use tools of war, figuratively speaking, that we older adults are too afraid to arm ourselves with.

**4. Senior citizens.** It is no secret that the largest chunk, 21 percent of all annual health care spending, was in the Medicare program in 2012.[81] This does not include Medicaid spending for dual eligible residents who may also be covered on Medicaid. They tend to be more physically frail than the rest of us. They require, in many instances, increasingly costly end-of-life care, which, even beyond the field of medicine, poses a whole other host of financial and ethical dilemmas.

Of course, seniors have a right to be cared for. Caring for the elderly is a moral duty. But seniors and their advocates also need to be active, reasoned voices on health care reform. They should help us tackle the hard issue of when to stop availing ourselves of medical procedures that prolong life but unequivocally fail to improve the quality of life.

**5. Families.** In an era when there are so many, diverse familial constructs, let's define "family" as a group of people residing in the same household, sharing expenses, resources and/or parenting duties. To amplify, in 2011, the US Census Bureau noted that 7.6 million couples lived together without being legally married, while married couples with children made up only 20% of all American households. However, 69% of all American children under 18 lived in two-parent homes, and 28% of American households of one person.[82]

And for all of those families that are not counted among the wealthy, health care is a big money matter. In fact, an overload of health care debt was the chief cause for 62% of bankruptcy filings by American

---

[81] Kaiser Family Foundation, 2012 Medicare Spending and Financing Fact Sheet, November 11, 2012; online at: http://kff.org/medicare/fact-sheet/medicare-spending-and-financing-fact-sheet/, (accessed July 24, 2014)

[82] United States Census Bureau, More Young Adults Are Living In Their Parent's Home Census Bureau Reports,   November 2, 2011; online at: https://www.census.gov/newsroom/releases/archives/families_households/cb11-183.html (accessed July 24, 2014)

families, according to a 2007 American Journal of Medicine article.[83] Further, in a 2010 survey presented by clearbankruptcy.com, medical expenses were the leading cause of personal bankruptcy at 42%. Job loss came in second at 22%.[84] Interestingly, if you remember that job loss often leads to loss of insurance and combine the two numbers, you get 64% which is very close to the 62% found in the JAMA study. These facts raise another troubling moral question: Even though more than 60% of Americans have health care insurance, many families suffer catastrophic financial loss when their breadwinners are waylaid by major illness. Why? American health care coverage is explicitly tied to one's ability to work. <u>This makes no sense.</u> When sickness or injury keeps an employee off the job it immediately puts that employee and all of his/her dependents' health care coverage at risk. If our health care system really worked, we would make provisions for waylaid breadwinners and their families. We would make it so that no American family grappling with major illness would needlessly fall into financial ruin.

**6. Employers and employees.** Employers and employees together, are doling out $600 to $650 billion a year to pay for insurance premiums. A 2011, Kaiser Family Foundation survey found that employer-sponsored health insurance premiums rose by 9% from the previous year; $5,049 to $5,429 for single person coverage. That same survey reported that employer premiums increased 113% between 2001 and 2011, while worker contributions had increased by 131% in that same time period.[85] Over this same period, statistics from the U.S. Bureau of

---

[83] Clear Bankruptcy.com, "Leading Causes of Bankruptcy"; online at: http://assetts.clearbankruptcy.com/infographics/leading-causes-ofbankruptcy.jpg (accessed July 24, 2014)

[84] Leading Causes of Bankruptcy, Clearbankruptcy.com; online at: http://assets.clearbankruptcy.com/infographics/leading-causes-of-bankruptcy.jpg, (accessed July 24, 2014)

[85] Henry J. Kaiser Family Foundation, Average Annual Premiums for Family Health Benefits Top $15,000 in 2011, Up 9 Percent, Substantially More than the Growth in Worker's Wages, Benchmark Employer Survey Finds, 2011 Employer Health Benefits Survey, September 27, 2011; online at: http://kff.org/private-insurance/press-

Labor show that employee wages increased by only 42%. *In short, our health insurance costs increased three times more than our salaries.* To be even more specific, if you salary increased by $5,000 over that decade, your health insurance premium probably increased by $15,000 over that same time period.

Obviously, employers are becoming less and less willing to pay increasing premiums and are passing that burden on to employees who are increasingly less able to bear that burden. This means even less take home pay for the American worker. In 2013, the average annual premiums for employer-sponsored health insurance were $5,884 for single coverage and $16,351 for family coverage. The single individual's insurance premium increased by 5% and the family premium by 4% over the 2012 average premiums.[86] During the same period workers' wages increased 1.8% and inflation increased 1.1%. Please note the reduction in the insurance premium in increase is post Obamacare. Traditionally, both employers and their employees have had very little leverage or legal recourse, despite the fact that these two groups are keeping insurance firms afloat and insurance CEOs very well compensated.

**7. You.** The individual, regardless of employment status, level of civic engagement, or degree of good health are the most important tool in the fight for health reform. It is the individual who can least afford to remain passive about a health care system in dire need of repair.

If, person by person, we each stood up, reinvested ourselves in ourselves, raised our separate voices and raised the bar for what we expect our government to do about health care, we could make more

---

release/average-annual-premiums-for-family-health-benefits/; (accessed July 24, 2014)
[86] Henry J. Kaiser Family Foundation in conjunction with the Health Research and Educational Trust, 2013 Employer Health Benefits Survey, August 20, 2013; online at: http://kff.org/report-section/2013-summary-of-findings/ (accessed July 24, 2014)

needed reform happen for sure. In fact, letting government ignore our interests and desires is a supremely un-American act. Ours is a great and proud country, steeped and formed out of citizen revolt, individual self-reliance, and pursuit of the common good:

- Our minimum wage was created through protest and citizen demand.

- Child protection laws and public education were created through protests and citizen demand.

- Voting rights for all were achieved through protest and citizen demand.

- Labor unions were created and worker rights were achieved through protest and citizen demand.

In short, most of the liberties, protections and best aspects of American life exist because you, the individual, wrote letters, picketed, marched, voted, and raised a ruckus. And you did so, in some cases, by putting your very lives on the line.

Fortunately for all of us there are simple things we can do that may have a larger impact than expected. To make it simple for myself, years ago I summarized tactics for social change under 3 P's: Petition, Phone Calls & Protest.

*Please do not underestimate clear courses of action such as letter-writing and petition campaigns, whether door-to-door or, even, online campaigns.* The Occupy Wall Street and 99% movements have gotten a lot of mileage out of online petitions and notices. As a result of protests launched through social media, Verizon backed off its surcharge for paying bills online. Stand-your-ground gun laws in states such as Arizona, Oklahoma and Florida (site of Trayvon Martin's tragic murder) have come under scrutiny.[87]    Petitions and resolutions are concrete proof of opinion on a topic.

Press your lawmakers to take firm legislative action by, among other means, presenting them with resolutions clearly stating your position.

*Rallies, marches and other public protests draw helpful, media coverage.*

I personally feel that the ultimate form of protest is divestment. The celebrated Montgomery Bus Boycott of the Civil Rights Movement was divestment at work. **Divestment from private for-profit health care corporations is certainly not out of the question.** Think big. Global divestment in South Africa's economy, which is credited with as crucial to bringing down racial apartheid, is probably the most noted contemporary example of the impact of stripping one's investment dollars from of a given market. We must all change our way of thinking and recognize that these heavily government supported health care industries are stealing our own money away from us. Hence, if they do not respond to our petitions, phone calls, and email then we should turn up the pressure and protest with our money and not just our mouths.

Many of you might be wondering, what you should demand in your petitions, phone calls and protests. I have listed my top five issues of concern below.

- **De-privatize American health care and remove private for-profit from our business model**. Our healthcare system is too

---

[87] Lizette Alvarez and Cara Buckley, "Zimmerman is Acquitted in Trayvon Martin Killing", New York Times, July 13, 2013; online at:
http://www.nytimes.com/2013/07/14/us/george-zimmerman-verdict-trayvon-martin.html?pagewanted=all&_r=0 (accessed July 25, 2014)

closely tied to our stock markets. Nearly seventy health care related companies were listed in the 2014 Fortune 1000 list. One should note that some of these companies were hospital systems like HCA and Community Health Systems.[88] (At minimum, place profit caps on health insurance, pharmaceuticals, hospitals, providers, medical supplies etc.)

- **Universalize health care** Basic care must be guaranteed across the board regardless of ability to pay. This is consistent with the US Constitution. If need be, we can stratify premiums so everyone except the extreme poor are paying something.
- **Transparency of cash flow, because we are being misled on a regular basis.** This happens because we do not know where our tax money and health premiums are being spent.
- **Ban lobbyists from using any form of cash towards politicians.** No campaign contributions, no paid educational trips. Our country has literally been auctioned off by private lobbyist money influencing the legislative process. We MUST put a stop to this.
- **Put Congress and the President into the same health insurance plan as everyone else.** A lot of the inertia in health care reform exists simply because no federal politician has to worry about health care coverage for the rest of their lives.

Please note that these are very simple changes. Opponents of these changes will lie to us and tell us that they are complicated and will destroy our country. They are not complicated and the only things these changes will destroy are the overinflated bank accounts of a select few, including several of our political leaders (as in Point No. 4). Feel free to use this sample resolution to make your voice heard.

---

[88] Modern Healthcare's "By the Numbers", December 23, 2013:4.

## Sample Resolution for Universal Health Care

*Whereas the US Constitution preamble reads: " **We the People**  of the United States, in Order to form a more perfect Union, establish Justice, insure domestic Tranquility, provide for the common defence, promote the general Welfare, and secure the Blessings of Liberty to ourselves and our Posterity, do ordain and establish this Constitution for the United States of America."*

*Whereas our Declaration of Independence states, "We hold these truths to be self-evident, that all men are created equal, that they are endowed by their Creator with certain unalienable Rights, that among these are Life, Liberty and the pursuit of Happiness."*

*Whereas it the right of the American people to demand a government that effects their safety, happiness, liberty, and health therefore be it resolved that:*

**It is un-American to treat police, fire safety, education, healthcare, and sanitation as private market commodities. They are public services that are citizens' rights guaranteed by our constitution and our tax payer base.**

**It is not the responsibility of the people to provide these services for themselves but that of the government of the United States in the same manner as our armed forces.**

**These services should be treated with the same priority and respect as the American Bill of Rights**

**As private citizen rights, police, fire safety, education, healthcare, and sanitation should not be governed by private corporations and for-profit ideology but the government with service efficiency, quality, and equality being the primary goals.**

*Having affirmed and uphold the aforementioned principles we the members of (your organization) resolve:*

*That is the ethical and constitutional responsibility of the US Congress to create & maintain legislation that guarantees every US citizen free and equal access to police, fire, education, healthcare, and sanitation.*

*The access and range of these services should not be limited or determined by citizen ability to pay.*

*Independent advisory boards consisting of local politicians, citizens, and clergy should be created to inspect and insure that these services are indeed being offered equally and fully.*

In addition to civil unrest and reclaiming our money in our health care, *we the people* also need to change. Here are some direct-care initiatives and other insights, many of them largely citizen-driven. Many of these initiatives will gain more of a spotlight as the Affordable Care Act proceeds toward full implementation and the questions for additional health care reform get hammered out.

**Health care cooperatives.** Plenty of medical conditions can be managed without the active involvement of a physician. Indeed, the growing scope-of-practice for nurse practitioners and physician assistants, people known as physician extenders, is partly due to doctor shortages in certain communities and regions of the country.

Several chronic conditions such as diabetes, hypertension, and cholesterol can be adequately managed with group visits. Specifically, as one example, a group of diabetics show up at the same time for check-ups, counseling, education, and peer support under the supervision of the "physician-extenders" I just noted. Patients in peer support groups tend to fare better. Please note: This does not mean completely removing physicians from the process. However, properly executed group visits, managed by non-physician staff, such as nurse practitioners, physician assistants, and nursing staff, actually allow for all involved to achieving comparable, quality outcomes at lower costs. Going this route means that, as a society, we must re-envision what a medical office looks like and entrust ourselves to qualified clinicians other than the doctor.

**Create your own insurance cooperatives.** In many ways, it remains to be seen which states will ultimately cooperate with the Affordable Care Act provisions to expand coverage of Medicaid, which, as previously noted, is the health care insurance for the poor that is paid for with federal and state funds. But why wait for the bureaucrats and politicians to decide the future of your health care? As a basic theory, insurance works by setting aside pooled resources to be spent on recovering from a catastrophe or accident, whether natural or manmade. Employers of all sizes could partner together to do this on their own, forming consortiums that contract with hospitals and physician groups.

It is easier than it sounds. In fact, some physicians have been doing a version of this through Independent Practice Associations (IPAs) that provide services to managed care organizations for a negotiated per-person fee, a fee-per-service basis, or for a flat fee. These physicians know there is strength in numbers. Several small businesses could contract with their own with IPAs, HMO's or other health networks to provide primary care coverage and specialty care for contracting business employees. Even allowing for required legal and administrative costs, employers who opt for IPAs could save significant money in comparison to their current health care plan costs.

Hospitals have been following suit because eight of the top-ten-revenue-producing U.S. health care systems in 2011, were also in the top-ten for the number of acute care hospitals. Further, five of those systems operated more than fifty acute care facilities.[89] One of the largest of these entities is the Roman Catholic Church, which controls four of the largest hospital systems in the United States. If you combine the revenues of these four Catholic operated healthcare systems; Ascension Health, Catholic Health Initiatives, Dignity Health (formerly Catholic Healthcare West), and Trinity Health, this becomes the second largest health care group in the nation, behind only the Veteran's Administration. In 2012, all four of these health systems were in the top ten criteria for revenue and the sheer number of facilities operated. Even those these health systems are separate they all must adhere to Catholic Health Care principles which come from Catholic Law and are ultimately under the guidance of the Pope.

One should note that the state-run medical exchanges in the Patient Protection and Affordable Care Act are actually a variation of this insurance cooperative idea. These exchanges remove the third-party payers and allows for private citizens and possibly even employers to buy coverage on more favorable terms.

**Live healthier.** That is the bottom line. Our biggest indicator of poor health has been obesity. The Centers for Disease Control and Prevention has been tracking obesity data for several years. The CDC defines obesity as a Body Mass Index or BMI >30 which is generally fits any adult who is more than 35lbs overweight. In 1991, there was not a single state where more than 20% of the population was obese. Sadly by 2006, 21 states had obesity rates greater than 21% and only 4 states had obesity rates that were less than 20%.[90]

---

[89] Beth Kutscher and Ashok Selvam, "Outward Bound, Survey Shows Hospital Systems, Even Those With Flat Volumes, Continue to Invest in Operations, Especially Outpatient Services," Modern Healthcare, June 4, 2012

[90] Robert Wood Johnson Foundation, F as in Fat: How Obesity Threatens Americas Future, Issue Report June 2010; online at:
http://healthyamericans.org/reports/obesity2010/Obesity2010Report.pdf
;(accessed July 24, 2014)

In spite of the supposed fitness craze of the 1980s and 1990s, modern America mostly has been eating itself into an early grave. Yes, some folks avidly watch what they eat and exercise. But although, on paper, Americans are living longer, we also are fatter and more sedentary than ever. This is especially the case with younger Americans.

In 2010, 12.5 million children aged 2 to 19 were categorized as obese. (Prevention)[91] Our youth, overall, also are less healthy. While rates of HIV-AIDS among adults have leveled off and held steady since 2001, they are rising among those aged 13 to 21. (Services, 2014)[92] After several years of decline, suicide amongst teens and college students has been increasing steadily since 2006 and is now the third leading cause of death amongst Americans aged 10 to 24. (Health, 2011)[93] But these facts are fodder for another book.

In spite of our vaunted health care technology, in 2010, three of the top 10 causes of death overall were completely preventable and were: suicide, pneumonia, and type II diabetes. Also preventable, and treatable, are heart disease, stroke, chronic lower respiratory disease, and a run-on list of accidents. Broadly speaking, as a culture and a people, we have got to take better care of ourselves. The following table represents my idea of improved general health care.

---

[91] Centers for Disease Control and Prevention, Prevalence of Childhood Obesity in the United States, 2011-2-12; online at:
http://healthyamericans.org/reports/obesity2010/Obesity2010Report.pdf ; (accessed July 24, 2014)
[92] U.S. Dept. Health and Human Services, Teens and HIV-Aids Epidemic, June 2012; online at: http://www.hhs.gov/ash/oah/news/e-updates/june-2012.html (accessed July 24, 2014)
[93] John Hopkins Bloomberg School of Public Health, Morbidity and Mortality Among Adolescents and Young Adults in the United States, Astra Zeneca Fact Sheet 2011; online at: http://www.jhsph.edu/research/centers-and-institutes/center-for-adolescent-health/az/_images/US%20Fact%20Sheet_FINAL.pdf ; (accessed July 24, 2014)

| Personal Care | Providers, not an institution or system, who continually engage, treat and mentor the patient. |
|---|---|
| Immunization/ Vaccines | They eradicate known diseases or keep known diseases at bay. |
| Dental | Dental coverage should not be separate from other aspects of medical coverage and care. Our teeth are not separate from our bodies. Oral health can influence overall health. This artificial separation creates more administrative costs and waste. |
| Mental Health | Virtually the same issue as dental. Americans should not have to pay special deductibles or process special paperwork for mental health services. |
| Sexual Health | STD's, unwanted pregnancies, rape are among reasons to guarantee this type of care, allowing women to make their own choices. |
| Screening | Cancer, tuberculosis, HIV, and glaucoma are just a few conditions where lives are saved or lengthened through screening and early detection. |
| Preventive Counseling | Patients should be able to engage physicians for mentoring and advice and it should still count as a billable visit. |
| Group Visits | Patients with chronic conditions fare better with group or peer support. |

**Accept our mortality.** In addition to living healthier, Americans have to become more comfortable with this one thing: We all will die. Many Americans, especially those in the legal and medical quality assurance communities, would do well to adjust their expectations and realize that fact. Health care is not and should not ever be painted as "immortality" care. Both the medical and legal communities should be more honest with the American public by admitting that even if the midst of technological "perfection," people still die. **As idealistic as it seems, the concept of "zero fail" is not practical for health care.**

**Sometimes the pills, procedures, tests, herbs and even prayers simply do not yield the desired results.** No one failed, nothing was missed, and nothing was done improperly. It was simply that person's time to leave this Earth.

None of these basic proposals are new. None are expensive. In fact, if guaranteed to every citizen, they would save money. The same is true of every intervention suggested in this book. None of them are exceptionally expensive but they would add significant access, quality, simplification and usability to our currently inaccessible, deficient and complex system.

Mark my words: Our leaders do few things unless we make those demands plain. So, yes, follow the 3 P's:

- Petition- sign them and write letters to officials
- Phone Calls- make them and send emails
- Protest- attend rallies and marches, protest with your money (divest)

Finally, let's all live healthier. Let's save our country. Let's save ourselves.

# Epilogue:

The idea for this book was birthed out of frustration. As a physician, I constantly encounter Americans of all socioeconomic backgrounds who are uninformed and believe totally false ideas as to what drives our American health care system. Once the ignorance became too much for me, I started writing. At first, I wrote to give myself hope that people would become informed before it was too late. Thus, I started writing imaginary answers to some of the questions I received. Before I knew it, I was thinking about what could and should be done about our overwhelming health care problem.

If we are going to conquer our health care system then we must embrace the fact that it is both an economic and moral plague that will destroy us if we do not correct it. Contrary to what our major media outlets report, abortion and end of life care are not the only major moral issues of American health care. When I talk with clinicians regarding troubling moral issues in healthcare, topics like mental health, preventive health, nutrition, lobbyists, tobacco and universal health care access are more prevalent. A whopping 25% of Americans suffer from mental illness with an estimated 1 in 5 of Americans on psychiatric medications.[94] Yet mental health is treated as a "special" circumstance by health insurers often demanding higher patient co-pays for services. Physicians are concerned about tobacco because nicotine is highly addictive but sold with less restriction than alcohol. In addition, a primary breakdown product of nicotine, N-Nitrosonornicotine (NNN)

---

[94] Richard A. Friedman, A Dry Pipeline for Psychiatric Drugs, New York Times, August, 19, 2013; online at http://www.nytimes.com/2013/08/20/health/a-dry-pipeline-for-psychiatric-drugs.html?_r=0. (accessed September 6, 2014)

has been shown to cause cancer in more than five human tissue types: breast, pancreas, lung, colon, larynx, and oral.[95] Heroin and cocaine have not been shown to cause cancer but are illegal substances. Why does tobacco and tobacco products remain legal?

Without a doubt there are many moral issues in American health care that receive little public attention; universal health care is probably the biggest issue. Right the now the discourse on universal health care has been framed and misshaped in the context of economics. Universal health care is not dangerous, hard, or outrageously costly. Universal health care is not free health care either. The primary issues to address when discussing universal health care should not be economics but morality and human decency.

Ironically, the principles of universal healthcare are already being advanced in our healthcare system. Medicare is proof of that, and aged Americans roundly laud that universal health care program. Through Medicare, CMS is already investigating possible quality and cost models such as variation reduction. This concept suggests that reducing the variability of physician habits in delivering care will also reduce costs. Universal health care will allow America to reduce variability in insurer practices, technology utilization, preventive medicine education, and of course, costs. Regardless, one must remember that the costs of healthcare corporate salaries, maintaining the arbitrary bureaucracy that denies many of us healthcare already outweigh what universal health care could cost us.

I sincerely doubt that we can realize the true benefits of reducing variability in costs and practice with universal health care unless we first change our primary motive. As long as we maintain a free market, capitalism-driven health care system, profit will remain the primary motive. Profit making behavior is what is killing our health care

---

[95] Neal L. Benowitz, Janne Hukkanen and Peyton Jacob, III, "Nicotine Chemisty, Metabolism, Kinetics and Biomarkers". Handbook of Experimental Pharmacology. 2009; (192): 29-60.

system. It is not our physicians, patients, or technology, but our motivation for profit, which causes daily conflicts of interest. Although the CEOs of various health care-related companies are easy targets, it is not fully their fault. As corporate leaders, it is their responsibility to maximize profits margins and generate dividends for shareholders. It is delusional for Americans to expect a fair and equitable health care system if it remains tied to our stock markets. Healthcare should not be a stock market commodity. We tolerate socialist practices, otherwise known as community resources in several areas of society such as police, fire, education, and sanitation. For both moral and economic reasons, health care should also be one of them.

# Bibliography

AFL-CIO. (2014, July 23). *Corporate Watch/Pay Watch*. Retrieved from AFL-CIO: http://www.aflcio.org/Corporate-Watch/Paywatch-Archive/CEO-Pay-and-You/CEO-Pay-by-Industry

Association of American Medical Colleges. (2011, October 1). 2011 Medical Student Loan Debt. (AAMc, Ed.) Retrieved July 24, 2014, from (https://www.aamc.org/download/309346/data/11debtfactcard.pdf)

Bish. *Healthcare Costs*. Tribune Review.

Bowman-Kruhm, M. (2003). *Margaret Mead: A Biography* (Vol. 1). CT, USA: Greenwood Press.

Buckley, L. A. (2013, July 14). Zimmerman is Acquitted inTrayvon Martin Killing. *New York Times* .

Bureau, U. S. (2011). *America's Families and Living Arrangements: 2011*. United States Census Bureau. U.S. government.

Bureau, U. S. (2012). *Labor Force Survey 2012*. United States Census Bureau.

Centers for Medicare and Medicaid. (2011). *National Health Expenditure Projections-2010 to 2020*. Centers for Medicare and Medicaid.

Centers for Medicare and Medicaid. *Shared Savings Program*. CMS Brief, Centers for Medicare and Medicaid, Baltimore.

Chapiatte. *Health Care Plan*. Political Cartoons.com.

Clear Bankruptcy.com. (2014, July 24). *Leading Causes of Bankruptcy*. Retrieved from Assetts.Clear Bankruptcy.com: http://assets.clearbankruptcy.com/infographics/leading-causes-of-bankruptcy.jpg

*Closing the Coverage Gap, Medicare Prescription Drugs Are Becoming More Affordable, Centers for Medicare and Medicaid*. (2014, February). Retrieved July

22, 2014, from Centers for Medicare and Medicaid.gov:
http://www.medicare.gov/pubs/pdf/11493.pdf

*Commonwealth of Massachusetts*. (2006, June 30). Retrieved July 22, 2014, from
malegislature.gov:
https://malegislature.gov/Laws/SessionLaws/Acts/2006/Chapter58

Congress, 1. (2010, March 26). Patient Protection and Affordable Care Act, Public
Law 111-148. Washington, D.C., USA. Retrieved July 22, 2014, from
http://www.gpo.gov/fdsys/pkg/PLAW-111publ148/pdf/PLAW-111publ148.pdf

(2014). *Congressional Budget Office.* Washington, D.C.: Congressional Budget
Office.

Congressional Health Care Caucus. (2013). *New 3.8% Medicare Tax on Unearned
Investment Income.* U.S. Congress, Health Care Caucus, Washington, D.C.

Contract Pharma.com. (2008, July 18). 2008 Top 20 Pharmaceutical Companies
Report. (G. Y. Roth, Ed.) USA. Retrieved July 24, 2014, from
http://www.contractpharma.com/issues/2008-07/view_features/2008-top-20-
pharmaceutical-companies-report/

Foundation, K. F. (2014). *Kaiser Foundation Annual Survey of Employer
Sponsored Health Benefits.* Menlo Park: Kaiser Family Foundation.

Foundation, R. W. (2010). *F As In Fat: How Obesity Threatens Americans Future.*
Henry J. Kaiser Family Foundation. Henry J. Kaiser Family Foundation.

Foundation.org, Henry J. Kaiser Family. (2011). *Health Reform Poll Finding.* Heny
J. Kaiser Family Foundation. Kaiser Family Foundation.

Frank, C. J. (2010, January). Ranking 37th-Measuring the Performance of the U.S.
Health Care System. *New England Journal of Medicine* , 98-99.

Fund, C. (2010). *U.S. Ranks Last on Health System Performance Measures.*
Commonwealth Fund. Washington., D.C.: Commonwealth Fund.

Garcia, J. (2013, October 2). Disney Offers Full-time Jobs to Part-timers Who Meet
Obamacare Threshold.

Gary Claxton, A. D. (2011). *Snapshots: Employer Health Insurance Costs and Worker Compensation.* Kaiser Family Foundation. The Henry J. Kaiser Family Foundation.

GFK Roper Public Affairs & Media. (2009). *Poll about Health Care Reform October 1st-5th.* GFK Custom Research of North America.

Greblov, L. S. (2005). *The Pharmaceutical Industry In The Global Economy.* Indianna University Kelly School of Business.

Hawkins, S. c. (2012). *A Survey of American Physicians.* The Physicians Foundation.org.

Health Level Seven International.org. (n.d.). *HL7 Standards:EHR Profiles.* Retrieved August 22, 2014, from HL7.org: http://www.hl7.org/implement/standards/product_section.cfm?section=4

Health Strategies Consulting, LLC. (2005). *Understanding the U.S. Pharmaceutical Supply Chain.* Kaiser Family Foundation.

Health, J. H. (2011). *Morbidity and Mortality Among Adolescents and Young Adults in the United States.* Johns Hopkins Bloomberg School of Public Health. Johns Hopkins Bloomberg School of Public Health.

Herzlinger, R. (2007). *Who Killed Health Care-America's $2 Trillion Dollar Medical Problem and the Consumer Driven Cure.* New York, U.S.A.: McGraw Hill.

*House Vote on HR 3590, 111th Conress.* (2010, March 21). Retrieved July 22, 2014, from Govtrack.us: https://www.govtrack.us/congress/votes/111-2010/h165

*Insure Kids Now.* (2014, July 23). Retrieved from Medicaid, Centers for Medicaid and Medicare: http://www.insurekidsnow.gov/medicaid/

Karen Davis, C. S. (2010). *Mirror Mirror on the Wall:How the Performance of the U.S. Health System Compares Internationally, 2010 Update.* Commonwealth Fund.

Karen Davis, K. S. (2014). *Mirror Mirror on the Wall: 2014 Update How the U.S. Health System Compares Internationally.* The Commonwealth Fund.

Kavilanz, P. (2013, April 8). *Small Business Doctors Driven to Bankruptcy.* Retrieved from CNN-Money: http://money.cnn.com/2013/04/08/smallbusiness/doctors-bankruptcy/

Kennedy, S. T. (2003). *Quality Affordable Health Care for All Americans.* National Institutes of Health. American Journal of Public Health.

Kim, E. (2012, June 28). *CNN Money.* Retrieved July 22, 2014, from CNN.com: http://money.cnn.com/2012/06/28/pf/taxes/tanning-tax/

Kolata, G. (2012, March 6). Knotty Callenges in Health Care Costs-An Interview with Victor Fuchs on Health Care Costs. *New York Times* . New York City. Retrieved July 21, 2014, from http://www.nytimes.com/2012/03/06/health/policy/an-interview-with-victor-fuchs-on-health-care-costs.html?module=Search&mabReward=relbia

Kolata, G. (2012, March 6). Knotty Challenges in Health Care Costs. *The New York Times* .

KR Levitt, H. L. (1996). Health Care Spending in 1994; Slowest in Decades. *Health Affairs* , *15* (2), 130-144.

Laura Snyder and Robin Rudowitz, with Eileen Ellis and Dennis Roberts. (2012). *Medicaid and the Uninsured.* White Paper.

Liptak, A. (2012, June 23). Supreme Court Upholds Health Care Law, 5-4 in a Victory for Obama. *New York Times*

Margaret Warner, P., Li Hui Chen, P., Diane M. Makuc, D. R., & and Arialdi M. Miniño, M. (20111). *Drug Poisoning Deaths in the United States-1980-2008.* U.S. Centers for Disease Control and Prevention. Centers for Disease Control and Prevention.

Matson. *Our Insurance Company Will Pay.* St. Louis Post-Dispatch.

McDonough, J. E. (2011). *Inside National Health Reform.* California, USA: University of California Press.

Medicaid, C. f. (n.d.). *CMS.gov/Open Payments-The Official Web Site for the Sunshine Act*. Retrieved August 22, 2014, from CMS.gov: http://www.cms.gov/Regulations-and-Guidance/Legislation/National-Physician-Payment-Transparency-Program/index.html

Merhar, C. (2014, January 16). *New Health Insurance Industry Taxes*. Retrieved July 22, 2014, from Zane Benefits.com: http://www.zanebenefits.com/blog/bid/273632/New-Health-Insurance-Industry-Taxes

Modern Health Care. (2013, December 2). IRS Creates Plan on Collecting Taxes to Pay for Affordable Care Act. *Cranes Detroit Business News* .

Mukherjee, S. (2013, June 21). *Insurers to Rebate Consumers 500 Million as a Result of Obamacare*. Retrieved July 23, 2014, from Think Progress.org: http://thinkprogress.org/health/2013/06/21/2194141/obamacare-big-insurers-overcharging/

National Conference of State Legislatures. (2014, June). Transparency and Disclosure of Health Costs and Provider Payments:State Actions. *2014 Update* .

Office, C. B. (2014). *Updated Estimates of the Effects of the Insurance Coverage Provisions of the Affordable Care Act, April 2014*. U.S. Congress, Congressional Budget Office-Joint Committe on Taxation. Washington, D.C.: U.S. Governement Office of .

Pear, S. G. (2010, March 23). Obama Signs Health Care Overhaul Bill, With a Flourish. *New York Times* .

Pfizer Pharmaceutical Company. (2007). *2007 Financial Report*. Pfizer.

Physicians for a National Health Plan. (2014, July 23). *Health Care Systems-Four Basic Models*. Retrieved from Physicians for a National Health Plan: http://www.pnhp.org/single_payer_resources/health_care_systems_four_basic_models.php

*PPACA Senate Vote on Senate Bill 396, 111th Congress*. (2009, December 24). Retrieved July 22, 2014, from Govtrack.us: https://www.govtrack.us/congress/votes/111-2009/s396

Prevention, C. f. (n.d.). *CDC.gov, Childhood Obesity Facts, Obesity Data-Childhood, 2011-2012*. Retrieved July 24, 2014, from Centers for Disease Control and Prevention.

Profiles , LLC. (2011, September 1). 2011-2012 Physician Salary Survey. *Profiles Database 2011-2012 Physician Salary Survey* . USA: Profilesdatabase.com. Retrieved July 24, 2014, from http://www.profilesdatabase.com/resources/2011-2012-physician-salary-survey

Quantia Inc. (2012). *Struggling Primary Physicians Could Undermined the Affordable Care Act*. Quantia Inc.

Researchers at the Kaiser Family Foundation, N. a. (Ed.). (2013, August 20). Retrieved July 6, 2014, from Kaiser Family Foundation.org: http://kff.org/report-section/2013-summary-of-findings/

Rosenow, K. (2012). *High Income Individuals to Pay Higher Medicare Taxes Starting in 2013*. Brief, Towers Watson.com.

Rosenthal, E. (2014, May 17). Medicine's Top Earners are not M.D.'s. *The New York Times* .

Saito, B. G. (2013, October). THE VALUE OF HEALTH AND WEALTH:ECONOMIC THEORY, ADMINISTRATION, AND Valuation Methods for Capping The Employer Sponsored Insurance Tax Exemption. *Harvard Law Journal* , 1-36.

Selvam, B. K. (2012, June 4). Outward Bound-Annual Survey Shows Health Systems, Even Those With Flat Volumes and Income, Continue to Invest in Operations, Especially Outpatient. *Modern Healthcare* , pp. 26-28.

Services, U. D. (2014, July 24). *Teens and the HIV/Aids Epidemic*. Retrieved from Office of Adolescent Health: http://www.hhs.gov/ash/oah/news/e-updates/june-2012.html

Singer, A. *No Exit*. Political Cartoons.com.

Squires, D. (2012). *Explaining High Health Care Spending in the United States: An International Comparison of Supply, Utilization, Prices, and Quality*. The

Commonwealth Fund, Issues in International Health Policy. The Commonwealth Fund.

State of New Jersey, Department of Labor. (2014, July 23). *Required Insurance for Employers*. Retrieved from New Jersey Department of Labor and Work Force Development: http://lwd.dol.state.nj.us/labor/wc/employer/require/insure_index.html

Steffie Woolhandler, M. M. (2003). Costs of Health Care Administration in the United States and Canada. *The New England Journal of Medicine* (N Eng J Med 2003:349:768-75), 768-775.

The Henry J. Kaiser Family Foundation.org. (2012). *Medicare Spending and Financing Fact Sheet*. The Henry J. Kaiser Family Foundation.org.

The Physicians Foundation. (2012). *Drivers of Health Care Costs-A Physicians Foundation Whitepaper*. The Physicians Foundation. The Physicians Foundation.

Trust, H. J. (2011, September 27). *Average Annual Premiums for Family Health Benefits Top $15,000 in 2011, Up 9 Percent, Substantially More than the Growth in Worker's Wages, Benchmark Employer Survey Finds*. Retrieved from Kaiser Family Foundation.org: http://kff.org/private-insurance/press-release/average-annual-premiums-for-family-health-benefits/

*U.S. Department of Health & Human Services*. (2010, March 23). Retrieved from Health and Human Services.gov: http://www.hhs.gov/healthcare/facts/timeline/index.html

*U.S.Department of Health & Human Services*. (2012, September 20). Retrieved July 22, 2014, from HHS.gov: http://www.hhs.gov/healthcare/facts/bystate/Making-a-Difference-National.html#PAGE

Unger, R. (2013, September 25). Wal-Mart Returning to Full-time Workers, Obamacare Not Such a Job Killer After All. *Forbes* .

Winter, R. E. (2013). *Unraveling U.S. Health Care-A Personal Guide*. Maryand, U.S.A.: Rowman & Littlefield.

Wolverton, M. *Big Health Insurance*. Cagle Cartoons.com.

Wyeth. (2008). *Wyeth Financial Report 2007.* Wyeth.

# Other Works Consulted

## Books

Kongstvedt, Peter. <u>The Managed Care Handbook.</u> 4th ed. Aspen Publishers, 2001.

Potter, Wendell. <u>Deadly Spin: An Insurance Company Insider Speaks out on how Corporate PR is killing Health Care and Deceiving Americans.</u> Bloomsbury Press, 2010.

Reid, T. R. <u>The Healing of America: A Global quest for better, cheaper and fairer health care.</u> Penguin Press, 2009.

Welch, H. Gilbert, Schwartz, Lisa M. and Woloshin, Steven. <u>Over diagnosed: Making People Sick in the Pursuit of Health.</u> Beacon Press, 2011.

## Periodicals

American Association for Justice. "The Ten Worst Insurance Companies in America: How They Raise Premiums, Deny Claims and refuse Insurance to Those Who Need it Most." n.p., n.d.

Bernstein, A, Hing, E., Moss AJ, Allen, KF, Siller, AR, and Tiggle, PB. "Healthcare in America: Trends in Utilization." Maryland: National Center for Health Statistics, 2003.

Cichon, Michael and Normand, Charles. "Between Beveridge and Bismarck-options for health care financing in central and eastern Europe." World Health Forum 15(1994):323-328.

Glick, Regina Marie "Highline Data Analysis Shows Revenue for Health Insurance Industry Groups Grew in 2007." <u>Reuters,</u> July 15, 2008. 27. Found online at: <u>http://www.reuters.com/article/2008/07/15/idUS187049+15-Jul-2008+PRN20080715 (accessed August 11, 2014)</u>

Institute of Medicine. Committee on Quality of Health Care in America. <u>Crossing the Quality Chasm: A new Health System for the 21st Century.</u> Washington D. C.: National Academy Press, 2001.

Kaiser/HRET surveys use the April-to-April time period, as do the sources in this and the following note. The inflation numbers are not seasonally adjusted. Bureau of Labor Statistics. Consumer Price Index - All Urban Consumers [Internet]. Washington (DC): Department of Labor; 2012 [cited 2013 June 16]. Found online at: http://data.bls.gov/timeseries/CUUR0000SA0?output_view=pct_1mth. (Accessed August 11, 2014)

Wage data are from the Bureau of Labor Statistics and based on the change in total average hourly earnings of production and nonsupervisory employees. Employment, hours, and earnings from the Current Employment Statistics survey [Internet]. Washington (DC): Department of Labor; 2013 [cited 201 June 16]. Found online at: http://data.bls.gov/timeseries/CES0500000008. (Accessed August 11, 2014)

Murphy, Sherry L, Xu, Jiaquan and Kochanek, Kenneth. Deaths: Preliminary Data for 2010- National Vital Statistics Reports. 60:4 (2012).

Medical Loss Ratio: Getting Your Money's Worth on Health Insurance. http://www.healthcare.gov/news/factsheets/2010/11/medical-loss-ratio.html (accessed August 11, 2014)

Premiums and Worker Contributions Among Workers Covered by Employer-Sponsored Coverage, 1999-2013; Henry J. Kaiser Family Foundation.org, and found online at: http://kff.org/interactive/premiums-and-worker-contributions (accessed August 11, 2014)

Somers, John and Keach, Richard. Employer-Sponsored Health Insurance, Costs, Offer Rates and Take-up Rates for Small Employers in the Private Sector, by Industry Classification, 2000 and 2003. Medical Expenditure Panel Survey, Statistical Brief #98. September 2005. Found online at: http://www.meps.ahrq.gov/mepsweb/data_files/publications/st98/stat98.pdf. (Accessed August 11, 2014)

Texiera, Ruy. "What the Public Really Wants on Health Care." The Century Foundation. n.p., n.d.

Winkler, Elizabeth, Basch, Peter and Cutler David. "3 Strategies for Reducing Health Care Administrative Costs." Center for American Progress, June 11, 2012.

www.ingramcontent.com/pod-product-compliance
Lightning Source LLC
Chambersburg PA
CBHW070539290526
45790CB00002B/571